magazine

ULTIMATE WORKOUT PLAN

By **Alistair McDonald**

Meal plans **Sion Colenso**
Photography **Tom Miles**
Design **Fanni Kosztolanyi**
Subeditor **Juliet Giles**
Model **Ben Kirby** @ **Premier**

With thanks to

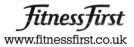

www.fitnessfirst.co.uk

For more information on Men's Fitness magazine, go to www.mensfitnessmagazine.co.uk.
To subscribe call 0844 844 0081.

Dennis Publishing

© Copyright Dennis Publishing Ltd. Licensed by Felden 2008

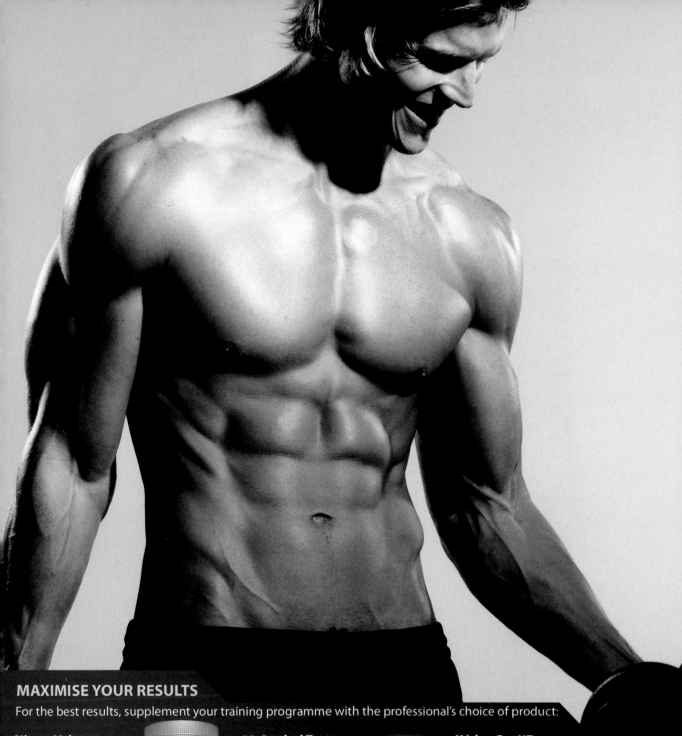

MAXIMISE YOUR RESULTS

For the best results, supplement your training programme with the professional's choice of product:

Nitrox Voltage

Nitrox Voltage is made up of a nitric oxide production stack, creatine absorption stack and an energy stack. The powerful combination of these stacks aids in the muscle generation process and creates explosive energy.

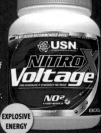

19-Anabol Testo

Developed to naturally increase your libido levels to the max. 19-Anabol Testo builds muscle and improves overall recovery from training. Add 19-Anabol Testo to your product combination strategy as your optimal, natural muscle-building supplement.

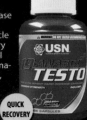

Xédra-Cut XT

2008 Xedra-Cut XT is USN's latest ground breaking weight-loss supplement, consisting of a synergistic blend of natural ingredients which have proven to assist in safe and effective weight-loss when used in combination with a training and eating plan.

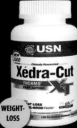

HARD MUSCLE MADE EASY!

Muscle Fuel Anabolic is your convenient, mega-loaded, all-in-one workout formula.

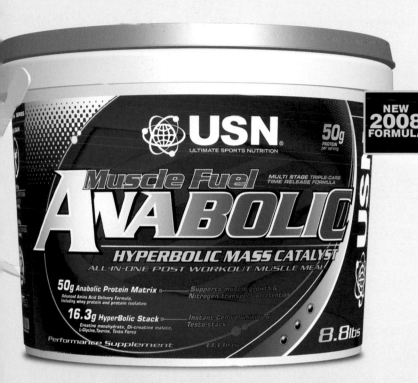

NEW 2008 FORMULA

Loaded with Creatine, Glutamine, an Anabolic Protein Matrix, T-boosters and an advanced amino acid delivery formula for rapid absorption, this is your optimum muscle supplement. Muscle Fuel Anabolic's great taste, convenient combination of active ingredients and rapid-absorption properties make this product perfect for individuals who are serious about building muscle mass.

Creatine
- Gain muscle, strength and size in just weeks
- Increase strength and energy during workouts
- Recover faster – train harder for longer

Glutamine
- Minimise muscle breakdown
- Improve protein metabolism
- Burn body fat and build new muscle
- Boost your immune system

T-boosters
- Build lean muscle
- Enhance your sex drive
- Increase energy
- Boost mood and memory
- Lower cholesterol and protect agains t heart disease

FACT FILE

If your aim is to increase lean muscle mass and reach your goals faster, you have to eat smart – up to six times per day! Hard training is not enough. Without the right nutritional building blocks it is impossible to build muscle. Fast Grow Anabolic is the perfect muscle-building meal replacement formula.

SPECIAL OFFER

Visit **www.usn.co.uk** and quote the promotion code in the specified field of the checkout section to receive **£5.00 OFF** your first purchase. Offer valid untill 28 02 2009.
CODE: MFTG01

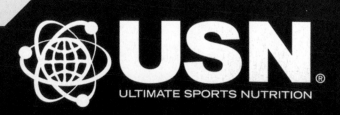

USN
ULTIMATE SPORTS NUTRITION

Tel: 0845 1800 556, Fax: 0845 1800 557, E-mail: info@usn.co.uk

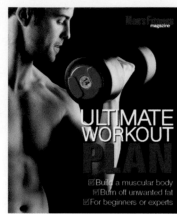

ULTIMATE WORKOUT PLAN CONTENTS

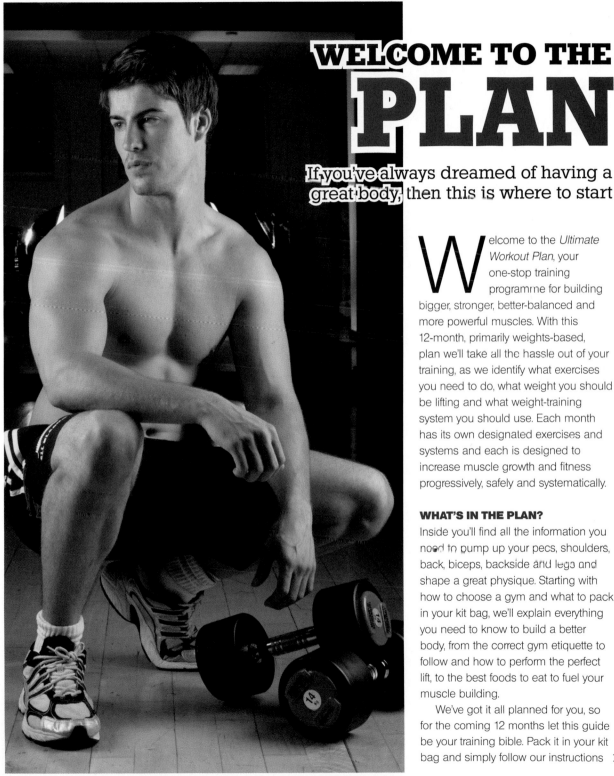

WELCOME TO THE
PLAN

If you've always dreamed of having a great body, then this is where to start

Welcome to the *Ultimate Workout Plan*, your one-stop training programme for building bigger, stronger, better-balanced and more powerful muscles. With this 12-month, primarily weights-based, plan we'll take all the hassle out of your training, as we identify what exercises you need to do, what weight you should be lifting and what weight-training system you should use. Each month has its own designated exercises and systems and each is designed to increase muscle growth and fitness progressively, safely and systematically.

WHAT'S IN THE PLAN?
Inside you'll find all the information you need to pump up your pecs, shoulders, back, biceps, backside and legs and shape a great physique. Starting with how to choose a gym and what to pack in your kit bag, we'll explain everything you need to know to build a better body, from the correct gym etiquette to follow and how to perform the perfect lift, to the best foods to eat to fuel your muscle building.

We've got it all planned for you, so for the coming 12 months let this guide be your training bible. Pack it in your kit bag and simply follow our instructions **»**

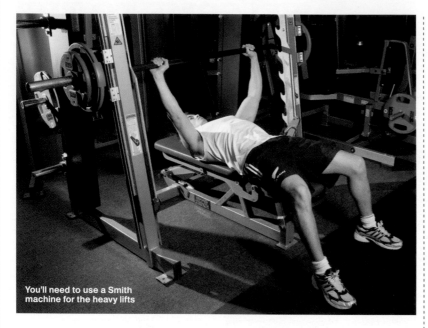

You'll need to use a Smith machine for the heavy lifts

burn unwanted fat and you'll also find that the more muscle you build the faster you'll burn that fat. For every 0.45kg of lean muscle gained you'll burn an extra 250-350 calories a week. That may not sound like a lot,

'It may seem pretty obvious that weight training is key to building muscle, but it's surprising how few men know how to use it effectively'

to the month-by-month workout programme (starting on p38). All you need do is record your progress in the training logs at the end of each month's workout and grow more muscle.

WHAT ELSE WILL YOU FIND?
As well as showing you the right exercises and training programmes we'll also show you how best to warm up for weights (and for cardiovascular training), how to minimise your injury risk, both by pre-training and gradually building up your training, and how to warm down. We've devised 12 simple meal plans that will provide all the nutrients and calories you need to feed your muscles. And to give your muscle building an extra boost we'll also tell you what supplements are worth spending your money on.

And because it's important that you vary your workout – to stimulate your muscle fibres – that's exactly what the

Ultimate Workout Plan will encourage you to do.

MAKING GAINS
If you follow the plan you should expect a month-by-month increase of around 0.5-1kg of lean muscle. After a couple of months your muscles will take on a more defined look, they'll be more toned, your physique will be better balanced and you'll feel great. A few months later and you'll be in peak, beach-posing condition.

Some men, notably those with athletic to large builds, will find it easier to pack on muscle than those with slighter frames. But the programme will work for everyone. Nutrition will be particularly important for slimmer men to pack in the healthy calories needed to increase muscle dimensions.

But even if your build is far from slim the programme will still work for you. Cardiovascular workouts will help you

but imagine how many calories you'll be incinerating when you pack on a couple of kilos of lean muscle.

GET IT RIGHT
It may seem pretty obvious that weight training is key to building muscle, but it's surprising how few men know how to use it effectively. Many assume the bench press on its own will give them the torso they crave and think that biceps curls are all they need to pump up their upper arms. Yes, these are important but there are other, better, exercises. Lots of men also make the mistake of neglecting their legs and backside. Bad idea. Aside from the fact you'll want muscled legs to balance your muscled upper body, you'll need those powerful legs to perform many of the upper-body exercises.

But perhaps the biggest mistake you could make is to assume that more is always better. Muscles are primarily made up of protein. Weight training breaks down this protein, creating microscopic tears in your muscle fibres, and it's in your downtime, when these fibres regenerate, that your muscles grow. So it's crucial that you factor in rest periods and recovery time and avoid doing extra workouts, which can halt your muscle growth.

THE CORE EXERCISES
In this plan we'll stick to core moves that are proven to build muscle. Mostly we've focused on compound exercises that work across a number of joints and involve large muscles. We have included some isolation exercises, such as biceps curls, but on their own these won't build muscle as effectively.

And although you might feel that we haven't included as many exercises as other programmes, you don't need to worry about being left feeling bored. We've included more than 60 exercises, and each month the programme will hit your body in a slightly different way, using different weight training systems to help keep both your mind and your muscles stimulated.

WANT A SIX-PACK?
Of course you do. Well, with the *Ultimate Workout Plan* you have every chance of getting one – once you've got rid of the fat from your gut. Specifically selected abdominal exercises will complement your weight training and encourage that slab of muscle down the front of your torso to make a rippling appearance. We've also designed specific cardiovascular routines that won't detract from your muscle-building weight training but will torch the fat that's hiding your abs. ■

Sample workout log

Workout log: month 1

See p41 for sets, reps and times

Theme: Getting ready to train **Date:** _12/10/08_
System: Simple sets, light weights
Speed of lift: 1:2
Rest. 0 minutes between sets and exercises

Exercise	Sets	Reps/Time	Weight
Bench tricep dip	2	10	N/A
Lunge	2	10	N/A
Chest press	2	10	15 kg each
Leg press	2	10	50 kg
Leg curl	2	10	20 kg
Seated dumb-bell shoulder press	2	10	10 kg each
Crunch	2	10	N/A
Plank	2	45 seconds	N/A
Swiss ball back extension	2	10	N/A

Sample Workout log

Log it as you do it...

Each month includes a workout log for you to record your progress. Simply photocopy the pages and use them to record the reps and times you achieve and the weights you lift for each workout. There's also space for you to record details of cardio workouts, such as the distance you've covered and power output generated.

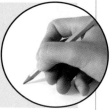

FREQUENTLY ASKED Questions

If you've got a training query the chances are we've got the answer...

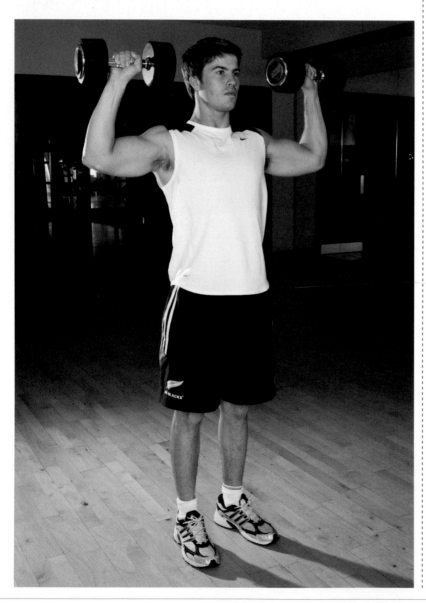

Q: Will weight training make me bulky?

A: This book will show you how to build muscle, but in an athletic way. You'll find workouts designed to boost your power and athleticism, as well as help you increase your muscle size. The aim is to develop an aesthetically pleasing and usable physique.

Q: Should I combine cardiovascular exercises with weight training?

A: Training the cardiovascular (aerobic) energy system and the strength, speed and power (anaerobic) energy system at the same time can result in one training method cancelling out the gains made by the other. The emphasis in this book is on weight training, but it is still important to do some cardiovascular work, so we have included some complementary cardiovascular workouts (see p28) that won't have a negative effect on your muscle building.

Q: Can I do the plan at home?

A: You'd need to have a good supply of weights in your garage as well as a proper bench and racks for squatting if you wanted to follow the plan at home. Instead, we recommend that you train in the right gym (see p12). In a gym you'll have all of the equipment that you need to complete the plan as effectively as possible.

Q: What if my gym doesn't have the right kit?

A: We'd be very surprised if you can't find a gym with the right kit. There are no unusual exercises in any of the workouts. You should be able to find a gym with the fixed and free weights and for the cardiovascular element you can lace up your trainers and go outside for a run or jump on your bike.

Q: Will I be able to take a holiday while I'm following the plan?

A: Of course. This is a training plan not a prison sentence. You'll be training three to four times a week, so you'll have plenty of rest days. The programme also includes recovery periods and months, so you could schedule your holidays for these times.

Q: I already weight train, should I start at the beginning of the plan?

A: If you have already developed a foundation of free weight training strength then you can start the programme at month three or four. But before you do that, it's important that you make sure you're proficient at all the lifts in the workouts and that you're ready to lift heavy weights in excess of 80 per cent of your one-rep maximum.

Q: I have a slim body shape, will I still gain muscle?

A: Yes. If you're naturally slim, eating the right food in the right quantities and taking supplements will be crucial (see page 22). You should also keep your cardiovascular work to a minimum. Your metabolism is probably already fast and so it won't need to be further revved up by cardiovascular work.

Q: How much muscle gain can I expect?

A: That's the million dollar question. As a guide, you can expect to add about 0.5-1kg per month, maybe more if you are completely new to weight training or you have the right genes.

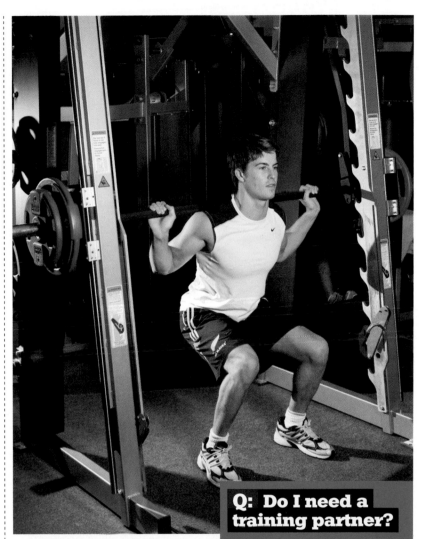

Q: If I'm progressing well should I add in extra workouts?

A: No. The plan is carefully structured to help you progressively build muscle. Extra workouts will reduce your chances of success because you need rest days when you're trying to build muscle. It's when you're not training that your body adapts to the workouts and builds stronger, larger and more powerful muscles. It can take up to 48 hours to recover from a tough workout.

Q: Do I need a training partner?

A: Ideally yes. A training partner will motivate and encourage you to train when you'd rather not go to the gym. He can also help you push yourself to the limit, which you'll need to do to build bigger muscles. Without one you'll need to use a Smith machine (above) when lifting heavy weights or peforming lifts such as bench presses. So, if you train alone, make sure the gym you choose has a Smith machine.

KNOW YOUR GYM!

What you need to check, do and take

Everything you need to know, to look and act like a pro in the gym

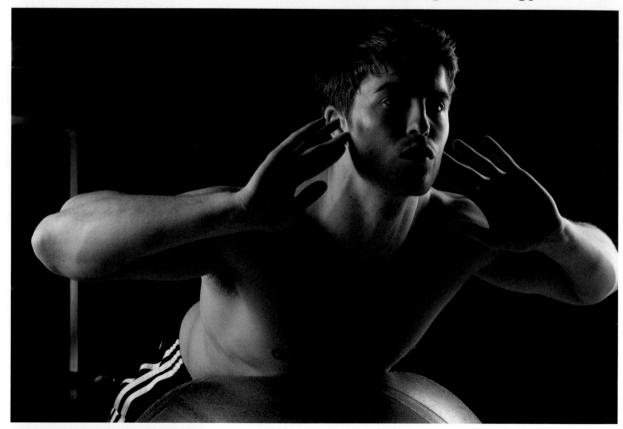

Key items to pack in your kit bag

■ Sweat pants and tracksuit top or sweatshirt.
■ Shorts.
■ Fitness training T-shirt or vest.
■ Trainers and socks.
■ Towel.
■ Drinks bottle containing a protein or energy-replacement drink. Or a protein bar (see p26).

LOCATION AND OPENING TIMES

Think about where and when you want to train. If you work long hours or have to do a lot of travelling to and from work then your best bet might be a gym close to your workplace.

CHECK OUT THE EQUIPMENT

Take a look round and see what kit they have. For the *Ultimate Workout Plan* in terms of fixed weights you'll need a leg curl, leg press, lat pull down, seated calf raise, which will invariably be plate loaded, chinning bar and cable crossover machine.

NOTE A Smith machine will be useful for lifting free weights – and, if you don't have a regular training partner, a necessity for lifting heavy weights. You should also make sure there are enough bars, benches, discs, dumb-bells and weight racks.

Cardiovascular equipment is less important for the plan, given its emphasis on weight training. But, if your gym has plenty of exercise bikes, treadmills and rowing machines then you'll be able to do all components of your workout under one roof – making your life easier.

GYM INSTRUCTORS
Check what qualifications and how much experience the instructors have. You'll need to be sure that they'll be

TIP
Keep an eye out for anyone training with heavy weights on his own and ask if he needs a spotter. If he says yes then you've found a way to get a set in between his – and possibly a new training partner.

able to offer you the right advice when you need expert help.

PEAK TIMES
Ask about the best times to train in terms of equipment availability and make sure these fit in with your own schedule. Some gyms will also you offer off-peak membership if you can train at less popular times, which could save you a lot of money.

WHO TRAINS THERE?
Traditional body-building type gyms feel a bit intimidating when you're just starting out. They shouldn't be if you stick to this plan, but don't allow your training to be affected by unsolicited and outdated training theory.

CHECK THE SMALL PRINT
A number of gyms, especially chains, will tie you into membership for a set period. Find out what the cancelation policy is and whether your membership will let you use other gyms in the chain. Don't pay for facilities you'll never use. ∎

Gym etiquette

Gyms tend to have lots of unwritten rules that can seem intimidating for newcomers. Top of this list can be interrupting other members' training to get onto the bench press or under the squat rack. You shouldn't be afraid to ask – though possibly not in the middle of a set. Politely ask them how long they're going to be or how many sets they've got left and whether you can jump in between. This way you can avoid standing around wasting time, and decide whether to move on to another exercise while you're waiting or substitute it with a similar move.

Other rules to remember:
- Always wipe down equipment after you've used it.
- Always return equipment to its 'home' after you've used it.

Weight trainers

When you start to lift heavier weights, using an X-trainer (or old school-type trainer with a relatively thin midsole) will be better and safer than a normal running shoe. This is because you need a stable lifting base and a running shoe, with a thick midsole that will compress, will not provide this. Weight lifters use shoes that are very stiff and offer ankle support. You don't need to go this far but a pair of X-trainers will do the job.

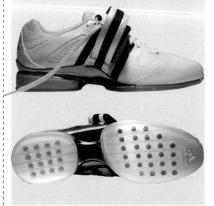

Weight belts and gloves

Weight belts
Don't use them unless you've previously injured your back and need the support. It's important you develop strength in your core (back and abs) to provide stability. The plank (see p43) and side plank (see p83) are key exercises for this.

Weight gloves
If you've never used Olympic bars and free weights before you'll

probably get sore palms, but don't be tempted to use gloves. In time your hands will harden, and lifting without gloves will also give you a better feel on the bar and produce better lifting.

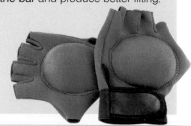

AVOIDING INJURY AND OVERTRAINING
Safety

Follow these simple safety steps to make sure you don't hurt yourself in the gym

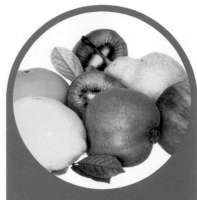

Rest and optimum nutrition will significantly reduce the chances of you overtraining

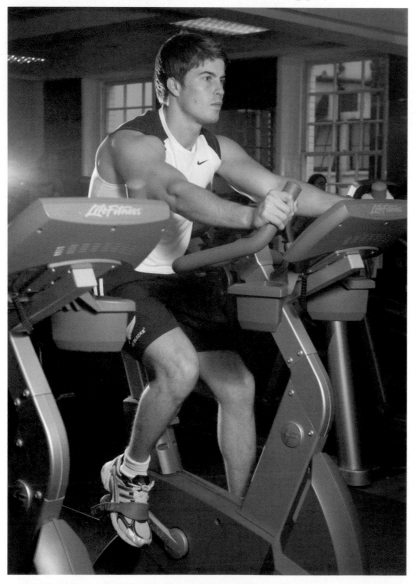

We've designed the *Ultimate Workout Plan* so you can safely build muscle progressively, but it's important you take note of the following guidelines:

1 Always underestimate what you think you can lift when first starting out on the plan, especially if you are new to weight training or you're returning after a long lay-off.

2 Learn correct lifting technique and follow our form tips on the workout pages and our lifting tips on p20.

3 Don't train when you are tired or ill (see overtraining signs, right).

4 Work with a spotter or use a Smith machine when lifting heavy weights.

5 Always check the condition of the equipment before you use it.

6 Put the collars on the bars – that's what they're there for.

7 Wear the right gear (see p12).

8 Don't be afraid to ask for advice from a suitably qualified and experienced trainer. You can't know everything.

9 Always warm up and warm down.

OVERTRAINING

Take a look at the overtraining symptoms listed below. If you think that two or more apply to you then you should think about taking some time off from your training programme. Normally three to four days should be enough to get you back on track, but when you return make sure you do so at a reduced intensity. If you continue to suffer from the symptoms (or they return quickly) take at least two weeks off. If the symptoms return again then there may be other causes and you should consult your GP.

'No matter how experienced you are it's crucial you warm up'

OVERTRAINING SYMPTOMS

- A lack of desire to train.
- Constantly feeling tired and listless.
- Decreased maximal heart rate.
- Greater susceptibility to illness – particularly in the throat and chest.
- Mood swings.
- Feeling anxious and stressed.
- An increase in resting heart rate (RHR). This should be taken a few minutes after waking; an increase above 'normal' can indicate that you have not fully recovered from your previous workouts or are suffering from stress.
- Sleep problems.
- Lack of appetite.

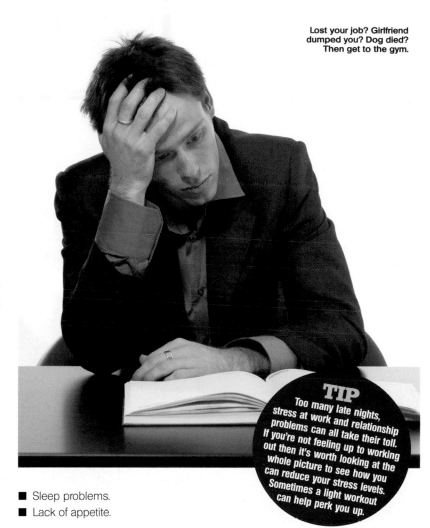

Lost your job? Girlfriend dumped you? Dog died? Then get to the gym.

TIP
Too many late nights, stress at work and relationship problems can all take their toll. If you're not feeling up to working out then it's worth looking at the whole picture to see how you can reduce your stress levels. Sometimes a light workout can help perk you up.

MUSCLE SORENESS

That 'ouch to the touch' feeling in your muscles, also known as delayed on-set muscle soreness (DOMS) is an inevitable consequence of trying to build bigger muscles, but it shouldn't be debilitating. It's most probably caused by the microscopic tears in your muscles that result from weight training. As these heal they produce bigger, stronger muscles – providing, of course, you are getting optimum rest and recovery – and it's this healing process that causes the soreness. If you haven't trained your muscles for some time then chances are you'll experience more soreness than someone who's been training for a while.

But no matter how experienced you are it's crucial that you warm up and warm down – as these processes will minimise muscle soreness. Vitamins A, C and E can also help to reduce the inflammatory responses associated with muscle soreness – as can a soak in a hot bath. ■

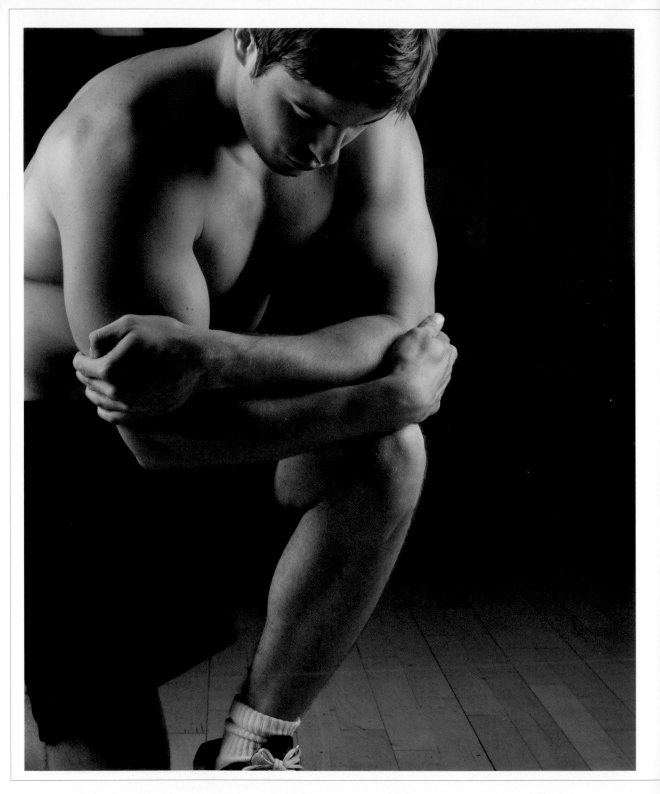

ALL YOU NEED TO KNOW ABOUT
Muscle building

If you understand the muscle building process you're more likely to enjoy your workouts and see great results

To get the most out of this plan you'll need to know where your muscles are and how they work. Over the page we've listed all the major muscle groups you'll be working, so you'll know what muscles you're targetting and you'll never confuse your lats with your traps again. And below we've included some tips on how to train your muscles to achieve maximum growth.

1 RING THE CHANGES
If you always do the same exercises in the same way your body will get used to the stimulus and your growth and strength will plateau. To avoid that you need to gradually increase the stress you place on your muscles. Progressively overloading your muscles, by using a heavier weight or increasing

the number of reps that you perform, will help them repair to become bigger and stronger than they were before.

2 KNOW YOUR HORMONES
Training helps kickstart your body into producing a number of anabolic hormones – most notably testosterone and growth hormone – which are responsible for muscle growth and repair. All the training workouts and meal plans we've included in the *Ultimate Workout Plan* have been designed to maximise this effect.

3 LEARN TO FAIL
To grow your muscles you need to push them beyond their comfort zone. Occasionally this will mean working a muscle to failure or to near failure. This means performing a lift to the point

NOTE

Muscles are made up of two types of fibres: slow and fast twitch. Slow twitch fibres use oxygen more efficiently and so are used during for endurance sports. Fast twitch fibres are better at generating short bursts of strength or speed and are called upon during heavy lifts.

MUSCLE FACT
There are over 600 muscles in the human body

where you can no longer maintain perfect form. You don't have to go to failure with every move. Certain sessions in the *Ultimate Workout Plan* are designed for you to focus on your lifting technique. In these workouts each rep must be explosive and performed with maximum effort to a 1:1 speed.

4 FIND A FRIEND
You can use a Smith machine for most moves but for the really heavy lifts you'll need to use a training partner or spotter. He must concentrate as much as you and only 'take the bar' at the point of failure. A training partner can also help keep you motivated and assist your forced reps – where you force out one or two more reps than you could achieve without help. ■

The key muscle movements

Muscles work differently depending on the direction in which you're working them:

■ Concentric moves
A concentric muscle action occurs when a muscle shortens as it contracts to create movement, such as when you lift a dumb-bell towards you in a biceps curl. Concentric

moves are the most common direction of effort for resistance and cardio exercise.

■ Eccentric moves
An eccentric muscle action is one that involves the lengthening of a muscle, such as when you lower a weight. Eccentric moves use more fast-twitch fibres.

Know your muscles

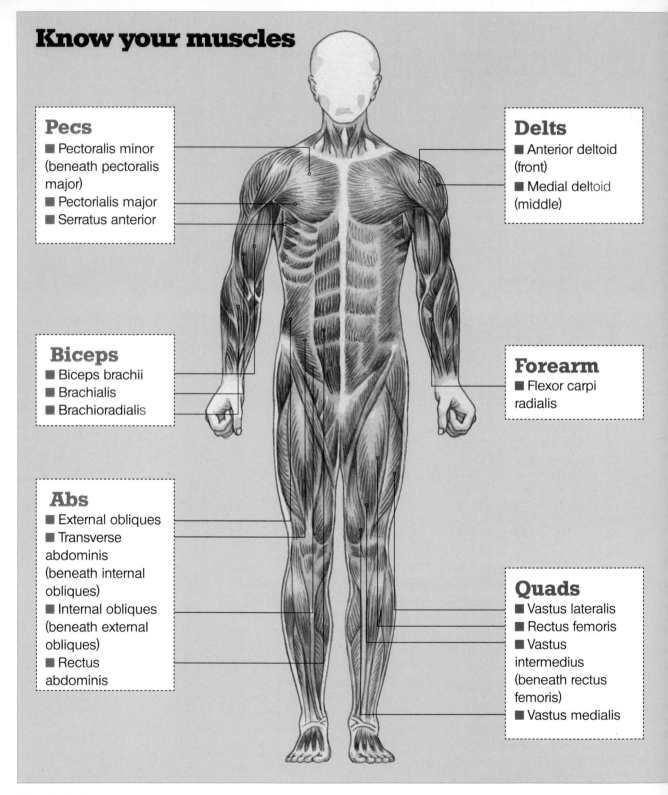

Pecs
■ Pectoralis minor
(beneath pectoralis
major)
■ Pectorialis major
■ Serratus anterior

Biceps
■ Biceps brachii
■ Brachialis
■ Brachioradialis

Abs
■ External obliques
■ Transverse
abdominis
(beneath internal
obliques)
■ Internal obliques
(beneath external
obliques)
■ Rectus
abdominis

Delts
■ Anterior deltoid
(front)
■ Medial deltoid
(middle)

Forearm
■ Flexor carpi
radialis

Quads
■ Vastus lateralis
■ Rectus femoris
■ Vastus
intermedius
(beneath rectus
femoris)
■ Vastus medialis

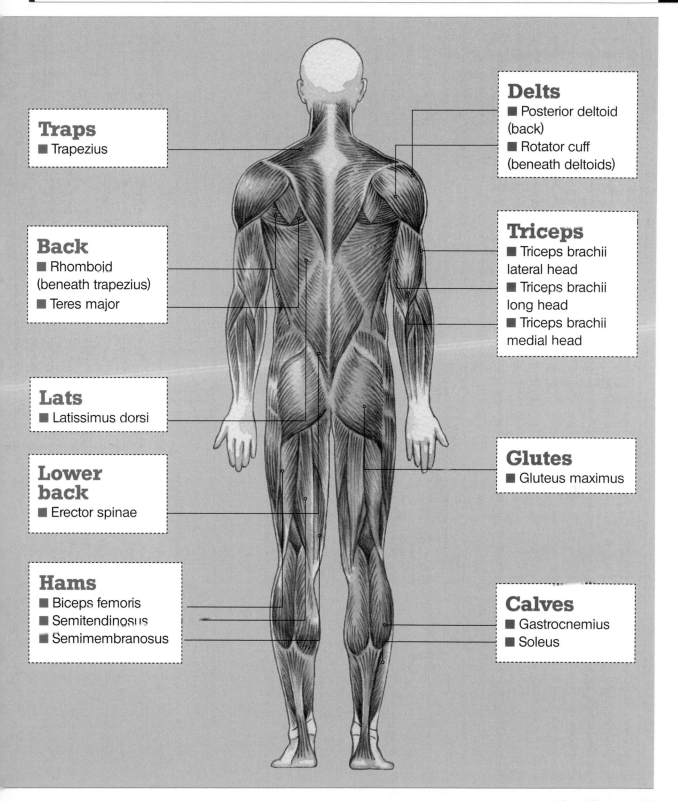

Traps
- ■ Trapezius

Back
- ■ Rhomboid (beneath trapezius)
- ■ Teres major

Lats
- ■ Latissimus dorsi

Lower back
- ■ Erector spinae

Hams
- ■ Biceps femoris
- ■ Semitendinosus
- ■ Semimembranosus

Delts
- ■ Posterior deltoid (back)
- ■ Rotator cuff (beneath deltoids)

Triceps
- ■ Triceps brachii lateral head
- ■ Triceps brachii long head
- ■ Triceps brachii medial head

Glutes
- ■ Gluteus maximus

Calves
- ■ Gastrocnemius
- ■ Soleus

12 STEPS TO THE...
Perfect lift

Follow the advice below to stay injury free and push your lifting ability up to new levels

How you lift a weight will make a huge difference to the results you see. If you lift with poor form, you're likely to get injured. Approach your workouts half heartedly and there's little chance you'll achieve your exercise goals. But if you focus properly and give maximum effort, you'll be pleased with the results. Keep these 12 tips in mind every time you lift and you'll further increase your odds of success.

1 Think about your workout for a few moments during the day before you do it. This will get you mentally ready to lift optimally.

2 Don't mess around in the gym. You're there to do a job. Mental focus is needed to optimise your lifting potential.

3 Check that the bar, collars or bench, and any other equipment is working properly before you lift.

4 Listening to music has been shown to boost lifting performance so crank up your MP3. But make sure your earphones and MP3 are well out of the way when you lift.

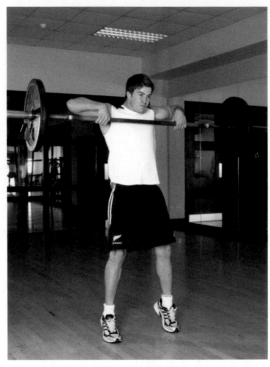

5 Make sure you are warmed up properly before you lift by following the pre-workout routine on pages 32-33.

6 Just before you complete your reps, focus and tell yourself that you will complete your set. Use 'self-talk'. Tell yourself that you are strong and powerful. This will gee you up. Also try to quickly run through in your mind what you are about to do. Visualise the lift being performed smoothly and at the designated speed.

7 Breathe in prior to each lift, brace your core and lift.

8 Brace your core, but maintain the natural curves of your spine throught the lift.

9 Breathe out when you lower the weight (complete the eccentric contraction). For the chest press reverse the breathing process so that you breath out prior to lifting and in as you press the weight. This will open the chest and allow you to work more of the muscle.

10 Make sure you work through the full range of movement required for the lift. This will ensure maximim muscle fibre recruitment and growth.

11 When the going gets tough don't sacrifice your form by, say, arching your back on the bench press because this could lead to injury.

12 Remain in the zone during your workout. Keep focussed and your muscles will respond.

Selected weight-training systems

	Simple sets	Drop sets	Supersets	Pre-exhaust	Split routine	Negatives (eccentric lifts)	Forced reps
Description	Each set contains the same number of reps. **For example,** 4 x 10 means four sets of ten reps.	This intense method of training begins with a heavy load. As many reps as possible are completed then some of the weight is removed. As many reps as possible are completed with the new weight before more weight is removed. This process continues for a designated number of sets.	Two exercises performed back-to-back without rest. These can either be non-competing supersets, such as chin-ups and squats, which work different body parts. Or they can be competing supersets, such as press-ups and bench presses, which work the same body parts.	You do an isolation exercise, such as a triceps extension followed by a compound move, such as a triceps dip.	Body regions, such as the legs, chest and shoulders are exercised during separate workouts. This enables maximum effort to be put into each body part.	These workouts emphasise the lowering (eccentric muscular contraction) phase of the lift. Take a slow five count as you lower the weight.	With the aid of a training partner you 'force' out 1 or 2 additional reps once you have reached failure.
Effects	Largely depends on the amount of weight lifted. If you lift medium-heavy and heavy weights you'll develop bigger muscles.	This system will have a serious anabolic effect and significantly overload your muscles.	Supersets are great at hitting muscle fibres and stimulating growth, particularly if you use meadium to heavy weights to target the same muscle group.	The first exercise reduces the targeted muscle's potential contribution to the second move. This means that the pre-exhausted muscle has to work harder during the compound exercise.	Split routines enable maximum mental and physical effort to be put into training each body part. They're also good because the system allows for relatively long periods of muscle recovery, and therefore growth, between workouts.	Super heavy weights (100-120 per cent of your 1RM), which you use during these lifts, will really hit your muscles hard, building fast twitch fibre.	This is a great way to stimulate muscle growth.
Comments	Despite their name simple sets are a very effective form of training.	This is an advanced system. At least 48 hours' recovery must be taken after these workouts. Protein consumption should begin immediately afterwards.	An advanced option.	Advanced exercise option because the execution of the compound exercise can be affected by the performance of the isolation move. As with drop sets, this system should be used sparingly	Get used to doing whole-body routines before you start tackling these workouts.	A training partner will normally be required to assist you throughout these workouts.	An advanced training option that requires considerable mental focus. Should be used sparingly but it's a good way to break through a weight training plateau.

ALL YOU NEED TO KNOW ABOUT
Basic nutrition

Use the advice in this section to eat the foods that will fuel your muscle building

Putting in some hard work at the gym is absolutely vital if you want to shed fat and pack on muscle. But so too is having a good diet. If you don't eat the right things at the right times you're not going to make the most of all that effort you put into working out. This section tells you everything you need to know about eating for more energy and for a better body.

The good news is that nutrition doesn't have to be complicated. In fact it's best when kept simple. And to make things even easier we've created 12 monthly meal plans that have been designed to provide you with the right number of calories and the ideal combination of carbohydrates, protein and fat to give you the best chance to build muscle. But we're not expecting you to stick rigidly to these plans, so over the next few pages we'll explain the basics for you to build your own meal plans.

CARBOHYDRATES

Carbohydrates are your body's preferred source of energy. Without them you'd struggle to get out of bed in the morning let alone complete any of the workouts in this book. Carbohydrates should always form the bulk of your meals but when your aim is to build

TABLE 1
Selected carbohydrates and their GI rating (out of 100)

Sugars		Boiled potato	56
Glucose	100	Banana	55
Sucrose	65	Sweetcorn	55
		Carrots	49
Bread, rice and pasta		Peas	48
Rice – *white*	87	Grapes	46
Rice – *brown*	76	Orange	44
Bread – *white*	70	Apple	38
Bread – *wholemeal*	69		
Pitta bread	57	**Dairy products**	
Spaghetti – *white*	41	Ice cream	61
Spaghetti – *brown*	37	Custard	43
Fettucine	32	Skimmed milk	32
		Full-fat milk	27
Breakfast cereals			
Cornflakes	84	**Pulses**	
Cheerios	74	Butter beans	31
Weetabix	69	Red kidney beans	27
Shredded wheat	67	Red lentils	26
Muesli	56	Soya beans	18
Porridge with water	42		
		Biscuits and snacks	
Fruit and vegetables		Rice cakes	85
Baked potato	85	Tortillas	72
Broad beans	79	Shortbread	64
Chips	75	Digestive biscuit	59
Watermelon	72	Chocolate	49
Pineapple	66	Muffin	44
Raisins	66	Peanuts	14

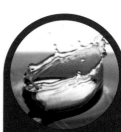

Drink up
You're going to sweat in the gym so you need to replace lost fluid with water. Make sure you rehydrate before you get thirsty. Take a water bottle to the gym and sip from it every few minutes, rather than glugging it all down in one go.

muscle they should make up around 60-65 per cent of your daily diet.

Carbohydrates can be either simple or complex (which isn't the same thing as refined or unrefined). Simple carbohydrates are basically sugars and will give you an instant energy boost, while complex carbohydrates are essentially starches, found in pasta, breads and vegetables, and will provide you with a slower release of energy.

Both types are broken down in your body into glucose, which is then absorbed by your cells and converted into energy. Any energy your body doesn't use is stored in your muscles (and liver) as glycogen. But this can only be stored in limited amounts and if you allow these glycogen stores to drop too low you'll suffer fatigue or, worse, your body will start to take proteins from other parts of your body, which could result in loss of muscle mass. After a workout your muscles are crying out for glycogen and can refuel their glycogen stores twice as fast as normal. So aim to eat a carb-based snack mixed with some protein within 45 minutes of finishing your last rep at the gym. A snack such as a bagel with cream cheese is a quick and tasty option.

The carbs you need immediately after a workout need to be mostly simple carbs with a high glycaemic index (GI). The GI, which ranges from 0-100, measures the speed at which energy is released from carbohydrates, with low GI foods releasing their energy more slowly than high GI foods. Understanding GI can help control your blood sugar levels, thus maintaining your energy levels and avoiding over-eating and optimally fuelling your muscle building. Table 1 (left) identifies

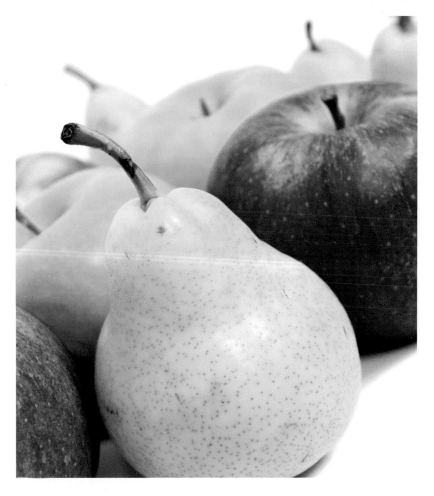

the glycaemic index of selected foods.

Although high GI carbs make an ideal pre- or post-workout snack you should try and base most of your meals around low GI carbs. Ideally these should be unrefined carbs, such as wholemeal bread or pasta, which not only give you a slow release of energy but are high in fibre. Aim to eat six small meals each day at regular intervals. This way you'll make sure that your glycogen levels are topped up and you'll prevent your body from breaking down the proteins you need.

PROTEIN

The one thing most men know about protein is that it helps build muscle. In fact muscles are essentially stored protein, which is needed for a variety of functions, including repairing tissue and transporting nutrients. But don't believe the myth that more protein automatically means more muscle. Aim to eat some protein with every meal but limit it to around 15-20 per cent of your daily diet. Most of our meal plans contain around 200g of protein per day. Eating more protein than this is pretty

TABLE 2
Micronutrients

Minerals

Twenty two, mainly metallic, minerals make up about four per cent of your body mass.

The main function of minerals is to balance and regulate your internal functions such as the maintenance of muscular contractions, the regulation of heart beat and nerve conduction.

Vitamins

Vitamins are crucial in facilitating energy release from food, but do not produce energy themselves. There are two types of vitamin:

■ Fat soluble (e.g. A,D,E and K), which are stored in the body.

■ Water soluble, which cannot be stored in the body and are found in fruit and vegetables (eg, B complex vitamins and vitamin C).

As with minerals, consuming excessive amounts (above the recommended daily intake) of vitamins will not enhance their metabolic contribution.

Antioxidants

Antioxidants include the vitamins A, C, E and beta-carotene and the mineral selenium. A diet rich in antioxidants can prevent cell damage, reduce LDL cholesterol and defend the body against age-related diseases, such as cancer and heart disease and can aid recovery from training.

useless because your body can't store the protein that you don't use.

Quality of protein is more important than quantity. Protein is made up of around 20 different amino acids, nine of which are called 'essential' because they can't be made in the body. Proteins that contain all nine of these essential amino acids are known as complete proteins and they also have a greater biological value (BV). This is a scale that measures how closely the protein's ratio of amino acids match the human body; the higher the BV, the better the protein will be for muscle growth and repair.

TABLE 3
Protein rating
(biological value)
of selected proteins

Protein source	Protein rating (biological value) out of 100
Eggs	100
Turkey	79
Fish	70
Lean beef	69
Peanuts	55

FAT

People sometimes assume that dietary fat is immediately converted to fat on the body. Not so. Eating more calories than you expend, whether they're from protein, carbohydrates or fat, is what causes the body to put down fat. Fat does, however, provide the most concentrated form of energy; it contains nine calories per gram, more than twice that of either protein or carbohydrates, so too much in your diet will quickly lead to weight gain. That doesn't mean you should banish all fat because it

serves crucial functions for the body, such as hormone metabolism, tissue structure and cushions organs, and transports the fat-soluble vitamins A, D, E and K. Ideally, fat should only make up around 25-30 per cent of your daily diet, but it's worth bearing in mind that not all fats are equal in terms of health:

THE GOOD **Unsaturated fats** come mostly from plant sources and are normally liquid at room temperature. They can be either monounsaturated or polyunsaturated, and are better for your heart health because they reduce levels of the 'bad' LDL cholesterol while raising levels of the 'good' HDL cholesterol, reducing your risk of atherosclerosis. One group of unsaturated fats are known as essential fatty acids because they can't be produced in the body and must be provided by food. Both omega 3 and omega 6 fall into this category. Omega 3, found in oily fish such as mackerel, is a fat you should try and get more of. It helps aid strength and aerobic training and helps protect the body from injury.

THE BAD **Saturated fats** are found mostly in animal products and are generally solid at room temperature. Saturated fats raise your LDL cholesterol and you should limit them to no more than 10 per cent of your total fat consumption.

THE UGLY **Trans-fatty acids (TFAs)** are commonly a by-product of the hydrogenation process that solidifies unsaturated fats. Trans fats increase your risk of heart disease and several other diseases. They're found largely in processed foods, such as cakes and biscuits and are often labelled as hydrogenated vegetable oils. Avoid them if you can.

TABLE 4 Vitamins and minerals

Selected vitamins and minerals, their muscle-building and fitness benefits and recommended daily intake amounts

Type	Biotin	Calcium	Iron	Zinc	Magnesium	Copper	Vitamin C
	B group vitamin	Mineral	Mineral	Mineral	Mineral	Mineral	Vitamin
Function	Assists conversion of food into energy and protein metabolism for muscle building.	Assists muscle contraction and hormonal signalling. Also important for strong bones.	Can assist aerobic exercise by promoting haemoglobin in oxygen-carrying red blood cells.	Important for metabolising proteins, carbohydrates and fats.	Boosts energy production and assists muscle contraction. Plays a role in blood sugar stabilisation and balances energy levels. Aids the production of new cells and muscle fibres.	Assists with soft tissue formation and serves an anti-oxidant role. Encourages the production of red blood cells and is useful for cardiovascular exercise.	Assists cell growth and repair. Aids absorption of iron from blood.
Recommended daily intake	10-200μg	1000mg	8.mg	9.5mg	300mg	1.2mg	40mg
Good sources	Egg yolk, nuts, oats and wholegrains, dried mixed fruit.	Dairy products, seafood, vegetables, flour, bread, pulses.	Liver, red meat, pasta and cereals, green leafy vegetables, eggs, prunes, wholegrains and dried fruit.	Lean meat and fish, eggs, whole grain cereals, dairy products, wholemeal breads and cereals.	Green leafy vegetables, fruit, unrefined wholegrains and wholegrain cereals, meat and dairy products.	Beef, liver, oysters, lamb, peanuts, baked beans, chick peas, wholemeal bread and whole grain cereals.	Fruit and vegetables, especially, strawberries, oranges, tomatoes, green peppers and baked potatoes.

ALL YOU NEED TO KNOW ABOUT

Supplements

You may find that using a supplement helps your training. Here's the essential information about the main varieties

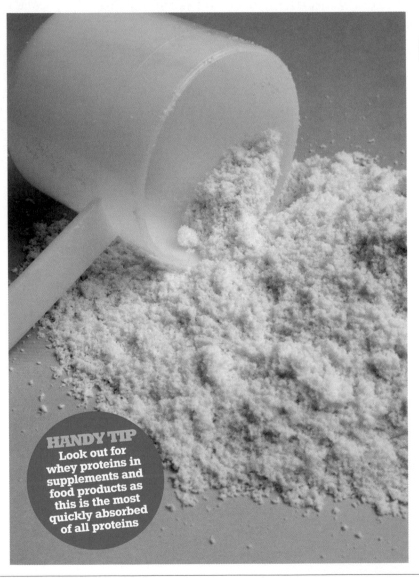

HANDY TIP
Look out for whey proteins in supplements and food products as this is the most quickly absorbed of all proteins

One question that we're asked more than any other on *Men's Fitness*, is: are supplements really necessary? Well, in theory, if you're following the rules outlined in the previous chapter, you shouldn't really need them. But, if you're struggling to get your 3,000 calories a day supplements can be useful.

CREATINE

If you're going to take one supplement, make it creatine. Research has backed up the claims that creatine can improve strength, power and muscle size. Creatine is produced naturally in the body from three amino acids (proteins). It's found in meat and fish, for example, but not in sufficient quantities to boost muscle building on its own, which is why you may need a supplement.

Creatine puts more of the high-energy releasing chemical compound phospho-creatine into your muscles. This allows you to train more intensely.

Take a loading dose, generally recommended to be 5g, four times a day for five days and then a maintenance dose of 2g a day for a month. Once the month is up you will get no further loading benefits and should cease use for a further month, before starting the process again.

PROTEIN SUPPLEMENTS

Weight training breaks down muscle protein. To make sure your muscles regenerate and grow, optimum protein replacement (and recovery) is needed to maintain and build bigger muscles. Aim to take on 1.5-1.7g of protein per kilogram of body weight per day.

WEIGHT GAIN SUPPLEMENTS

If you want to maximise your potential to build muscle then you'll probably

'Creatine can improve strength, power and muscle size'

need to increase your calorie consumption to provide both energy for your training and sufficient muscle building materials (unless you are overweight, in which case a careful balancing act between calories in and calories out is required). This is because your normal calorific consumption won't

be enough to achieve your workout goals. In this instance a weight gain supplement can be useful, because of the hundreds of additional calories it packs. These usually combine quick digesting whey protein with equally quick energy releasing carbs. Some also contain specific fats that are calorie dense, good energy suppliers and less likely to be turned into body fat.

HMB (BETA-HYDROXY BETA-METHYLBUTYRATE)

HMB is produced in the body from proteins. Among the few foods to contain HMB are grapefruit and catfish. HMB can increase muscle size and strength and decrease body fat. Research also indicates that it can reduce muscle soreness. The recommended dose is 3g a day.

FAT BURNERS

Fat burning products are designed to elevate the body's metabolic rate and mobilise fat as an energy source.

CHECK YOUR SUPPLEMENTS

You should always check the supplement product labelling and buy from a reputable supplier. Most products are designed for those with lactose intolerance. If in doubt about using a supplement contact your doctor.

Many contain the stimulants caffeine and guarana. We recommend that fat burners are avoided because regular training and a balanced diet will up your metabolic rate by as much as 20 per cent, which will help you to burn fat naturally.

GLUTAMINE

Glutamine is found in muscle cells and is crucial for optimum immune system functioning. It's made from amino acids.

Glutamine should be taken immediately after exercise and again within two hours after your initial intake. However, research into glutamine's claimed benefits is at present much less consistent compared to that produced for creatine, for example.

NOTE The recommended glutamine dose is 2-3g per day (although with this supplement recommendations very greatly). If you are taking a protein supplement then you will invariably be increasing your body's glutamine stores in any case (look either for glutamine or glutamic acid as part of the product's content).

Surround your workout with protein

Recent research has highlighted the importance of consuming protein prior to resistance training to prime muscles for maximum growth during recovery. It has been well known for quite some time that supplementing post exercise will increase the rate of protein synthesis and speed up the recovery and the growth of new, stronger muscle tissue.

Look for protein supplements containing whey, as this is the most quickly absorbed of all proteins.

NOTE Excessive consumption of protein (and too little carbohydrate) can lead to digestive problems, nausea, bad breath, osteoporosis and a lack of essential micro-nutrients being absorbed into the body.

Cardio training

Some people will tell you that cardio and weight training don't mix.
We say differently, but you do have to get the balance right...

Normally, building muscle and cardiovascular training don't sit well together. They're like the yin and yang of fitness training. Both have their benefits but mix them together and your body gets confused because you're training two different physiological energy systems: the aerobic and the anaerobic.

Aerobic training strengthens your heart and lungs (cardiovascular system), and is great for torching unwanted fat and improving your general fitness levels, but it's not so great when you're trying to build muscle. Too much cardio training can actually break down your muscles and replace your bulky fast-twitch muscle with the leaner slow-twitch kind. Anaerobic weight training, on the other hand, will build muscle but won't have the health benefits of cardio. Luckily, if you follow these three simple tips, and stick to workouts in this book, you can have the best of both worlds.

CARDIO TRAINING TIPS

1 Don't train too much

Unless you're overweight when you start the plan, don't do any more than 20 minutes of cardio training in one session after the first three months. Any more than this and you may start to compromise your muscle gains.

If you do need to shed some pounds, then for the first three months you should do three cardio workouts a week rather than just two. This additional workout should be a steady paced effort of no more than 45 minutes after your weights workout, or on a rest day in weeks with just two workouts. Once you've got your weight down to a healthy BMI (see p37) follow the cardio training sessions as normal.

2 Complement your training

Because they train the anaerobic energy system – the same system targeted by weight training – short and sharp interval workouts will complement weight training more easily than simply going for a long run.

These short, stop-start, fast workouts are what we've called complementary interval training workouts throughout the *Ultimate Workout Plan*. They look tough, but if you have a reasonable level of cardiovascular fitness – you're able to run easily for 40 minutes and feel relatively fresh – you should have no trouble in completing them.

Unless otherwise stated you should perform all of the cardio workouts listed once a week, normally after your weights workout (see cardio FAQs p31).

3 Train to recover

If you are feeling particularly sore after a weights workout then a steady 20-minute run or cycle can flush out some of the waste products that have accumulated and speed up your recovery for your next workout.

Looking good

All the cardio workouts included in this book have been designed to complement your weight training and improve the way your body looks.
The complementary interval training workouts involve both fast movements and the need to overcome moderate-to-heavy resistance, which means they'll develop muscle mass in a way that's not too dissimilar to weight training. These workouts will also help elevate your metabolic rate, which when combined with all your other workouts will ensure you are naturally burning more calories, torching your unwanted fat and increasing your lean muscle mass. All of which adds up to a muscular, athletic physique you're going to be proud to show off on the beach.

A Stair sprint

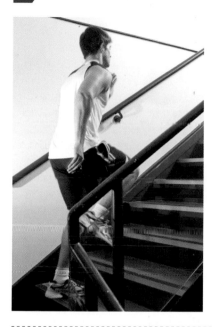

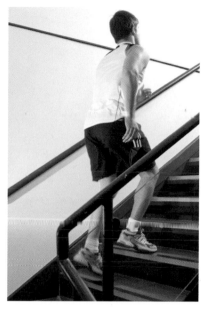

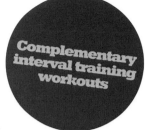

Complementary interval training workouts

■ To perform this exercise effectively you'll need to find somewhere you can run safely that has more than 30 steps. Run up the stairs for 10-15 seconds, turn around and walk slowly back down and repeat 10 times. This workout will add power to your thighs and upper body as you pump your arms back and forwards in time with your legs to boost your speed.

B Exercise bike sprint

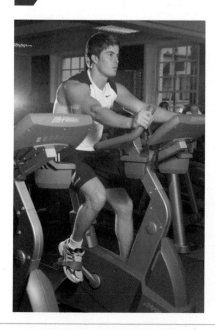

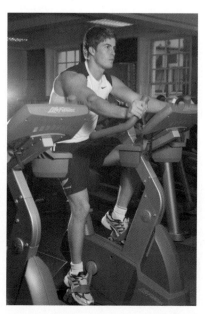

■ Adjust the bike so that you are pedalling against a tough resistance. Perform a 30 second sprint and take 90 seconds recovery. Repeat 6-8 times. If your legs really start to burn, then extend the recovery period or stop the session. Doing this will keep the emphasis of the workout on power and strength, rather than endurance. You can record in your log the power output you achieve on each rep, or the distance you complete, from the bike's display.

C▶ Running sprint

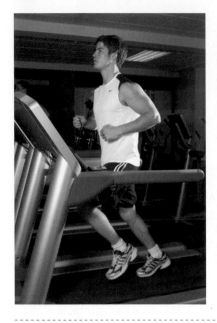 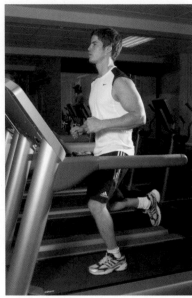

■ If you have access to a running track, or dry flat grass, then sprints are a great way to boost your muscle building. Every time your foot hits the ground you will have to overcome around three times your body weight. And your foot will only be in contact with the ground for about a tenth of a second. Generating this amount of power and with such frequency in the weights room would be impossible. Perform 6 sets of 30m sprints from a standing start. With a complete recovery between each set.

NOTE You can use a treadmill but your workout will not be as effective – sprint on a very fast belt speed for 30 seconds.

D▶ Rowing power stroke

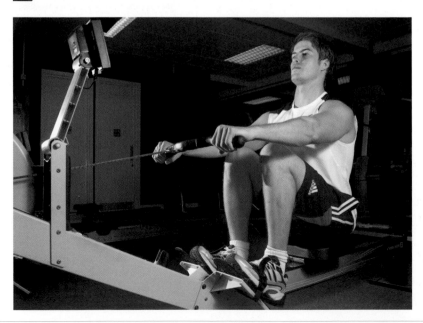

■ Do 10 sets of 10 strokes at maximum effort on a rowing machine, performing 60 seconds of easy-paced rowing between sets. If the machine allows, set it so you can read your power output on each stroke and record the average of each set of 10 strokes. Make sure you have good rowing technique before you do this session. As with the cycling workout, if your legs start to really burn increase your recovery between efforts or cut short the session.

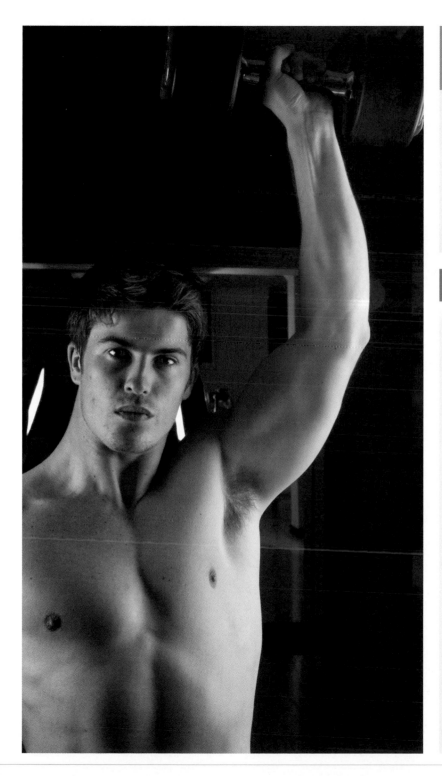

Keep your muscle protein in your muscles

Too much cardio exercise can compromise your muscle building by shrinking your muscles. Protein can be used by the body as an energy source – regular and prolonged cardiovascular workouts will start to rob your muscles of their protein content. That's why marathon runners are stick thin and sprinters are muscle-bound power houses.

Specific cardio FAQs

1 **Why do your steady pace cardiovascular training after your weights workouts?**
Very simply it's because you want to put quality energy and prime mental focus into your weight training. If your mind and muscles are tired then your focus will be compromised and your muscle growth will be less than optimum.

2 **When should I perform the complementary workouts, before or after my weights?**
You can perform the rowing and cycling workouts after your weight training. However, you should give yourself about 10 minutes to recover from your weights workout before you tackle any cardio workout. Warm-up on the relevant machine with five minutes easy paced activity. You'll need to be fresh for the sprints and stair sprints workouts, so save these for a separate training day when you're not performing a weights workout.

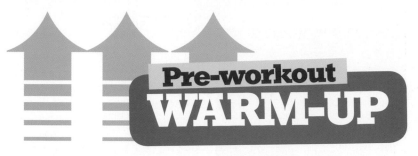

Pre-workout WARM-UP

Get your muscles ready for the hard work to come with this pre-workout warm-up

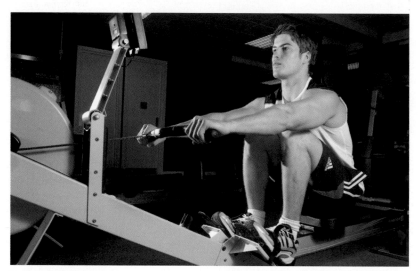

WHY WARM UP?

Lots of men don't like to stretch, preferring instead to get straight into their workouts. But while you might think 10-20 minutes spent warming up is a waste of your valuable gym time, in the long run it could save you wasting several days laid up at home because of injury. Just a few minutes of light cardiovascular work will make your heart beat faster, which pumps oxygen and nutrients to your muscles, and raises your core temperature. Warm muscles are more elastic, so you can work them through a greater range of motion with less chance of injury. Once your muscles are warm you can move on to some dynamic moves (see opposite) to target the muscles directly.

HOW TO WARM UP
1 For weights workouts
a) Do three to five minutes of moderate cardio activity, such as rowing or running on the treadmill.
b) Perform some dynamic movements, such as walking lunges, marching on the spot, arm and leg swings, calf raises and squat jumps – see opposite. Build up the speed of these exercises gradually. These movements will prime your muscles for explosive action. Take your time and recover between sets.
c) Perform a very light set of 10 reps of the weights exercise you are going to attempt. Take a minute or two to recover before completing your designated workout.

2 For cardio workouts
Follow parts 'a' and 'b' of the weights warm-up, but use the same cardio equipment you're going to use for the main part of your workout. Also, if you're planning to do either the stair sprint workout (p29) or the running sprint workout (p30) do 4 progressively faster runs over 40m, taking recovering fully between efforts.

DYNAMIC MOVES
The dynamic movements on the opposite page will help boost your weight training. They stimulate the nervous system and help activate your fast-twitch fibres. Performing the squat jump exercise, for example, should allow you to lift heavier leg weights for about 30 minutes afterwards. And if your want to achieve a similar effect for your arms then you could perform medicine ball throws. You do this by holding a medicine ball at chest height and either throwing it to a partner a couple of metres in front of you or by throwing it against a wall. Pass and catch the ball as fast as you can for 3 sets of 20 reps.

1 Walking lunge

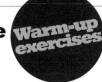
Warm-up exercises

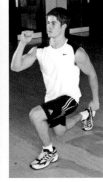
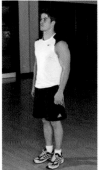

■ **Key tip:**
Step forward
into a lunge
and, in a fluid
motion, step
through with
your back leg
and repeat the
move.
Do: 5 x 10

4 Arm swings

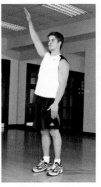
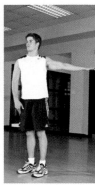

■ **Key tip:** Swing
your arm forwards
for ten reps, then
backwards for ten
reps. Swap sides
and repeat then
do the same with
both arms at the
same time.
Do: 10 reps in
each direction.

2 Marching on the spot

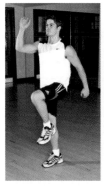
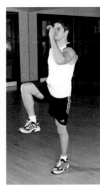

■ **Key tip:** Stay
tall and try to
co-ordinate your
opposite arm
and leg.
Do: 5 x 20. Build
up speed.

5 Leg swings

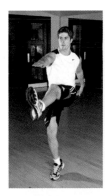
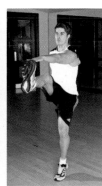

■ **Key tip:** Relax
and swing your
leg forwards and
backwards, pivoting
at the hip. Swing
your arm to meet
your foot and
gradually build up
speed and range of
movement.
Do: 2 x 10 on

3 Calf raises

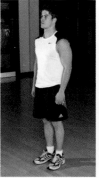
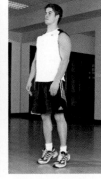

■ **Key tip:**
Lift your ankles as
far off the ground
as you can. Lift
to a 1 count
and lower to a 3
count. **Do:** 4 x 10

6 Squat jumps

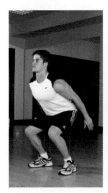
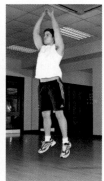

■ **Key tip:**
Sink into a squat
and, assisted by
momentum from
swinging your
arms, explode up
off the ground.
Land as lightly
as you can and
repeat the move.
Do: 3 x 4

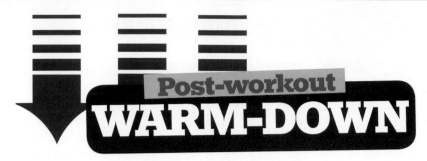

Post-workout
WARM-DOWN

Get your warm-down right and you'll be primed and ready for your next muscle-building workout

WHY WARM DOWN?

You probably think that once you've completed a gruelling workout the only thing left to do is relax in a hot bath and then flop on a sofa. Well you'd be wrong. Warming down is as important as warming up, for two good reasons:

It helps flush out lactic acid

A tough workout can lead to a build up of lactic acid in your muscles. Lactate is produced throughout the day as your body breaks down glucose, but during normal exercise, such as walking, your muscle cells get enough oxygen for them to use energy from other sources.

But, during very intense anaerobic workouts, where demand for energy is high but oxygen levels limited, lactate can accumulate to a point where it can no longer be re-absorbed and re-used to create energy. At this point lactate changes to lactic acid and you start to get that burning sensation in your muscles. A warm down will increase blood flow and start to flush the muscles of lactic acid, reducing the potential for soreness and stiffness.

It assists protein growth

Warming down will also speed up the growth of new muscle-building protein in your recovery periods by flushing your muscles with nutrient-rich blood supplies. Stretching assists this process and helps to elongate muscles. Weight training can shorten muscle fibres and, over time, this can lead to poor posture. Stretching can help you avoid this.

HOW TO WARM DOWN

Part A Easy paced cardio work

After your workout do 5 minutes, at an easy intensity, of any cardio exercise, such as cycling or running. If you've just finished a cardio workout, however, always use the same piece of cardio equipment you've been using for your workout, so that you're targeting the same muscles you've just worked.

Part B Stretching

After you have finished your gentle cardio work, walk around for a couple of minutes and shake out your arms and legs. Then perform each of the stretches on the page opposite 3 times and hold each one for 10 seconds. Keep warm while you stretch.

Nutrition as part of your warm-down (and warm-up)

Protein

When you work out you increase the blood flow that carries nutrients, including amino acids (see p23), to your muscles. By eating a protein-rich snack before and after your workout you'll ensure that your muscle cells get the optimum delivery of amino acids for muscle growth.

This will also create a positive hormonal response in your body by stimulating growth hormone and testosterone release, which will boost your muscle building. Ideally, you should aim to take on 20g protein before your workout and 20-40g after your workout.

A protein bar can be a good way to refuel because you can stash them in your gym bag. The best contain around 21g of whey protein, along with carbohydrate and other nutrients.

Carbohydrate

In the two hours immediately after a workout your muscles can replenish their glycogen stores (see p22) one and a half times more quickly, so this is the ideal time for a carbohydrate snack. Opt for high GI carbs (see p22), such as raisins that will give you a quick release of energy. Ideally, you should eat 1g of carbs for every kilogramme of body weight.

Stretching exercises

Use held stretches, rather than the dynamic movements you used in your warm up. Relax and don't try to force the stretch or bounce to gain an extra stretch.

1 Shoulder stretch

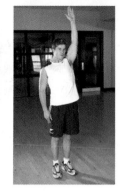

■ Stand tall and lift your arms, one at a time, up by your ear. Press the arm back, but don't bend forward.

2 Chest stretch

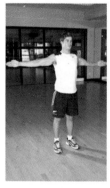

■ Stretch your arms out in front of your chest, with your palms facing each other. Take both arms out to the sides as far as you can, keeping them parallel to the ground throughout.

3 Abs stretch

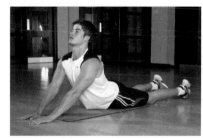

■ Lie on your front with hands in line with shoulders. Push up to lift your torso from the floor. Keep hips in contact with the floor.

4 Glute stretch

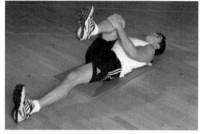

■ Lie on your back. Clasp one knee and pull back as far as it will go. Keep your other leg straight and your shoulders on the floor.

5 Hamstring stretch

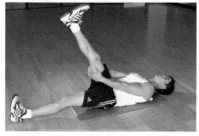

■ Lie on your back. Clasp the back of one thigh and pull that leg back as far as it will go. Keep the other leg straight.

6 Quadriceps stretch

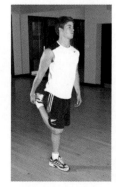

■ Stand on one leg and pull the other up toward your backside, pointing your knee towards the ground.

7 Calf stretch

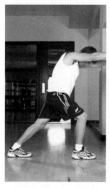

■ Stand at arms' length from a wall and place both hands on the wall. Take one foot back and press your heel into the floor.

Test yourself

Keep yourself on track for success by measuring your progress with these seven self tests

You'll need to stay motivated if you're going to complete all the workouts. And nothing will motivate you more than quantifying how much your fitness and strength are improving. You can complete the tests as often as you like but you may want to do them at the end of every month. Whenever you do them, make sure you are feeling fresh before you start the test.

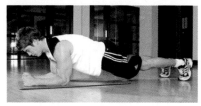

TEST 1: PLANK ENDURANCE

Tests: Core strength.

You'll see once you get started on the workouts that the plank (and variations on the plank) form a key part of the programme. It's also an excellent indication of your core strength.

How to perform: Simply see how long you can hold the plank position. When you begin to sag or seriously shake then it is time to stop. You must use the same indicator each time otherwise you'll skew your results.

How do you score?

Average:	30-45 seconds
Good:	45-60 seconds
Very Good:	60-90 seconds
Excellent:	90-120 seconds

Superhuman:	120+ seconds

TEST 2: HAMSTRING STRETCH

Tests: Hamstring and hip flexibility.

How to perform: Lie on your back and pull one leg into your chest by holding behind the thigh. Keep your other leg and your back on the floor (see p35). Once you have settled, pull your leg gently further back while keeping it straight. You'll need to gauge the angle of your leg to the floor so a training partner might come in handy.

How do you score?

Average:	70°
Good:	90°
Very good:	100°
Excellent:	110°
Stretch Armstrong:	120°+

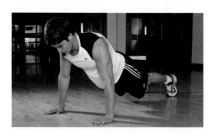

TEST 3: PRESS-UP TEST

Tests: Upper-body muscular endurance. Although the *Ultimate Workout Plan* focuses on building muscle, your local muscular endurance will increase across the programme. This is because – everything else being equal – a stronger muscle is more enduring than a weaker one. So even without specifically training for press-up endurance you should find that your ability to perform lots of reps increases over the months of the programme.

How to perform: Simply perform as many strict form press-ups (see p59) as you can without stopping.

How do you score?

Average:	20-30
Good:	31-50
Very good:	51-60
Excellent:	61-70
Duracell Bunny:	71+

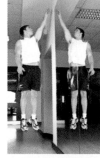

TEST 4: VERTICAL JUMP

Tests: Explosive leg power. The *Ultimate Workout Plan* will help boost your muscles' ability to express power. Not only is a larger muscle able to perform more reps, it will also be capable of expressing more power. So, as you progress through the plan you should find that your jump power, as well as other dynamic movement, increases.

Some of the workouts in this guide – especially those using the 1:1 speed of lift – will help you to develop real dynamic power. They'll 'teach' your muscles to recoil and contract with great speed, as they would do when you're jumping and sprinting.

How to perform: Stand next to a wall and stretch up with your arm nearest to the wall. Use chalk to mark the highest point of your reach. Step slightly away from the wall. Bend your knees and jump as high as you can marking the wall with the chalk. Take three attempts, and measure the distance between your jump marks and your standing mark. Record your best score.

How do you score?

Average:	35-45cm
Good:	45-55cm
Very good:	55-60cm
Excellent:	60-65cm
Rocket Man:	65cm+

TEST 5: STRENGTH

Tests: Muscular strength.
Once you've followed the *Ultimate Workout Plan* for five months you can test your one-repetition maximum (1RM) – that's the maximum you could lift on a specific exercise once. These sessions are very strenuous and should be completed when you are feeling fresh. You should also have a training partner on hand to spot for you.

NOTE If you are an experienced weight trainer you can test your 1RMs at an earlier stage.

How to perform: Do a few light weight warm-up lifts, take a minute to get in the zone and attempt to lift more than your previous 1RM max on the bar/machine. You will get a feel during your session as to whether you are 'ready' for it or not. Listen to your body and don't push to excess. You will only be able to go for

a couple of 1RMs in a workout – bench and squat, for example.

The following scores for the bench press and the squat have been provided as guidelines only. They should be seen as a starting point for your quest for increased strength. As you progress through the months of the *Ultimate Workout Plan*, you should significantly improve your 1RMs.

Bench press 1RM

Average:	50-70% of body weight
Good:	70-80% of body weight
Very good:	80-90% of body weight
Excellent:	90-100% of body weight
Arnie:	100%+ of body weight

Barbell squat to thighs parallel to the ground

Average:	80-90% of body weight
Good:	90-100% of body weight
Very good:	100-120% of body weight
Excellent:	120-130% of body weight
Arnie:	130%+ of body weight

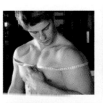

TEST 6: MEASURE UP

Measures: muscle growth.
This is not so much a test as a tool to measure your muscle-building progress. You simply measure your muscles and record your size increases.

How to perform: Simply use a tape measure to measure your:

Biceps/triceps: when you are contracting them with a 90° elbow bend.

Chest/back/shoulders: from the centre (widest) point of your outer deltoids across the centre of the pecs.

Chest/back: under your armpits and across the widest point of your chest.

Thighs: at their widest point

Calf muscles: at their widest point

TEST 7: BODY MASS INDEX (BMI)

Tests: Body composition.
Again this is less of a test and more of a tool to measure your body fat. It's not helpful to carry this test out on a monthly basis as it won't distinguish between extra weight carried as fat and extra weight in the form of muscle. It is, however, a good test to perform before you begin the programme to see if you need to shift some fat before you start to pack on muscle. The cardio exercises (p28) will help torch fat and boost your metabolism. Building extra muscle will also help you burn calories faster.

How to perform: Divide your weight in kilograms by your height in metres squared and compare your result to the BMI reference scores below:

BMI Reference Scores

Underweight:	Below 20 BMI
Ideal weight:	20-25 BMI
Overweight:	26-30 BMI
Obese:	31-40 BMI
Clinically obese:	40+ BMI

The Workouts

It's time to step out of the science class and get into the gym

Now you understand the theory behind the workouts it's time to put the theory into practice. We've divided the workout into 12 specific monthly routines. Each month has a theme that builds on the strength, size and fitness developed in the previous month. Every month we've included an illustrated description of how to perform each exercise, and a handy reference box to explain how many sets and reps you should perform of each. Unless otherwise stated you should perform all of the exercises in all of your workouts, leaving the core exercises to the end. We've also included a selection of cardio workouts (see p29-30) that have been specifically designed to complement your weight training.

UNDERSTANDING THE WORKOUTS

At the start of every month we've included a workout summary box. At the top of the left-hand column you'll see we've listed the system used. This will be explained in more detail in that

month's introduction, but you'll find a brief description of all the systems featured in the book in the table on page 21. We've also included in this column the weight you should be using along with a list of the exercises and the number and type of cardio sessions you should perform each week. Where the number of sets or reps differs from the norm we've listed those next to the individual exercise.

The right-hand column lists the number of workouts you'll complete each week, along with the number of sets and reps. So, in Month 1, Week 1 you'll see three workouts labelled a, b and c. This means you should perform three workouts that week, leaving at least one day's rest between workouts.

Most weeks will include three workouts, but some will include only two. These are easy weeks and are included to promote muscle growth and mental recovery. Don't be tempted to add in any extra workouts, or miss any out. If you find the progressions too difficult then cut back on the number of sets and reps.

Sets and repetitions (reps)

The number of times you perform each exercise in the workout will vary from workout to workout and week to week

Month theme and aims

■ Each month also has an introduction that will explain in more detail all the key features. We've given each month a theme and an aim. This is to give you an idea of what you should have achieved by the end of the month. For example, Month 1's theme is 'Getting ready to train', and its aim is to 'pre-train the body, using bodyweight, fixed-weight machines and dumb-bells', and that's exactly what you'll be doing.

and these are listed next to each workout. So in Month 1, Week 1, Workout a, you'll see the figure: 2 x 10. This means you perform 2 sets of 10 repetitions of each exercise. So, for example, with the triceps dip you'll lower and raise your body 10 times before taking a 2-minute rest and then performing the exercise 10 more times for your second set. For unilateral exercises that work one limb at a time, such as the lunge, you need to perform the stated number of repetions for each arm or leg. The length of time you'll rest between sets and exercises will vary from month to month.

WEIGHT LOADINGS

The loading of the weights you use is as important as the number of sets and repetions. To get your fast-twitch fibres growing you need to lift medium, medium-heavy and heavy weights. Light weights won't hit your muscles hard enough or in the right way to stimulate growth. For most months you'll see the weight you should be using listed alongside the system. But in some months, where the weight varies from workout to workout, we've listed the weight alongside each workout.

What constitutes a light or medium weight will vary, depending on your individual level of strength and fitness. The best way to gauge the weight is as a percentage of your one-repetition maximum (1RM). This refers to the maximum amount you could lift once on a specific exercise. You can estimate your 1RM by performing ten repetitions with your top weight with perfect form,

'Each month has a theme that builds on the strength, size and fitness developed in the previous month'

and then multiplying this weight in kilogrammes by 1.33 for your upper-body moves and 1.54 for lower-body moves. Once you have this figure you can then work out how heavy a weight in kilogrammes you should be lifting by using the following percentages:

■ **Light weight: less than 65 per cent 1RM** – a weight you could lift 15-30 times before failure.

■ **Medium weight: 65-75 per cent 1RM** – a weight you could lift seven to 12 times before failure.

■ **Medium-heavy weight: 75-85 per cent 1RM** – a weight you could lift five to seven times before failure.

■ **Heavy weight: 85-100 per cent 1RM** – a weight you could lift no more than five times.

■ **Super-heavy weight: 100-120 per cent 1RM** – a weight you would be unable to lift, but could lower (eccentrically) one to three times.

SPEED OF LIFT

Varying the speed at which you lift and lower the weight is a great way to keep challenging your muscles. We've used three speeds: 1:2, 1:5 and 1:1. The first figure refers to lifting (concentric) speed and the second the lowering (eccentric) speed. So for a 1:2 lift you would lift to a count of one and lower to a count of two. Each speed has its benefits:
1:2 This is the basic weight-training speed, which can be used with all

loadings. This speed will have a medium-high effect on stimulating your muscle building hormones.
1:5 This speed puts more emphasis on the lowering (eccentric) phase of a move and so targets more fast-twitch fibres. It works best with medium-heavy, heavy and super heavy weights, and will have a high stimulatory effect on your muscle-building hormones.
1:1 This explosive speed will develop size and power and have a significant hormonal effect as you move the weights as fast – but as safely – as you can. It recruits significant amounts of fast-twitch muscle fibre.

CHART YOUR PROGRESS

Each month has its own workout log for you to record the actual weight you lift and the reps you complete. We've also included space for you to record your cardio workouts. Make a note of which workouts you've completed and, where applicable, the distance and power outputs of your reps. There's also space for you to record your progress in the self tests outlined on pages 36-37.

The workout comments section is for you to record any relevant information on how your workout went. If your workout was a great success say so. If not then record that as well. Working out why things went well or badly will help you to improve for your next workout.

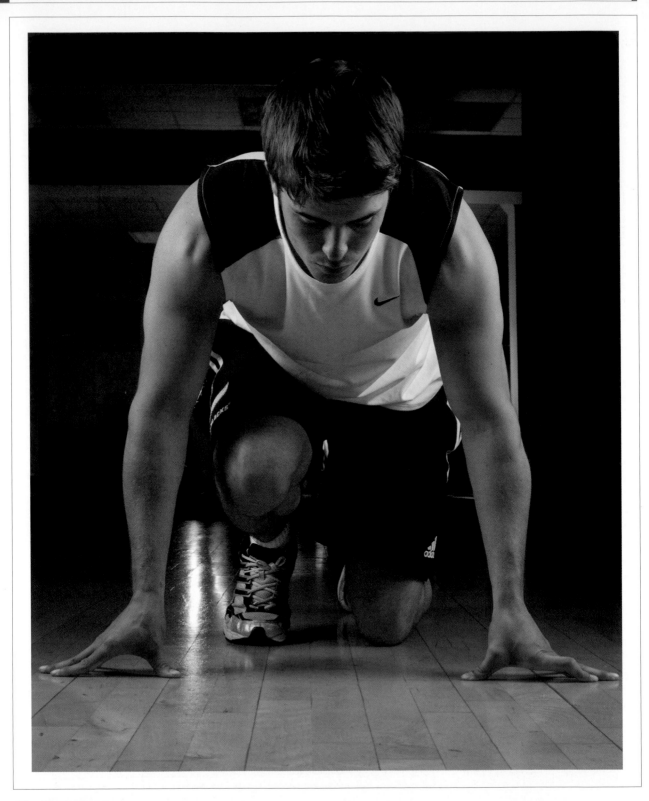

Ultimate Workout Plan
MONTH 1

Month one is all about getting your body used to working out and lifting weights safely. You'll see we've included a number of bodyweight exercises. These will help develop some preliminary strength to prepare you for the more strenuous training in later months. And with the plank, crunch and Swiss ball back extension exercises we're also putting the emphasis on the core. This is because your core plays such a vital role in lifting weights that it's important you fully condition it against potential injury.

We've included one free-weight exercise – the seated dumb-bell shoulder press – which you need to perform using light weights. This will help develop the shoulder stability you'll need to perform the overhead exercises in later months. The cardiovascular sessions are designed to provide a base of fitness, which will boost your recovery during your weights workouts in future. Depending on your fitness levels these workouts should take up to 30 minutes of steady-state effort.

Core exercises

Leave your core exercise to the end of your workouts. You don't want to fatigue this area before you perform the weights exercises, as your abs and back need to be able to contribute fully to your lifts.

Month 1:

AIM to pre-train the body, using bodyweight, fixed-weight machines and dumb-bells

System
Simple sets, light weight

Bodyweight
Bench triceps dip
Lunge

For the lunge, perform the required number of sets for each leg.

Free weights
Seated dumb-bell shoulder press

Fixed weights
Chest press
Leg press
Leg curl

Core
Crunch
Plank
Swiss ball back extension

For the plank start with 5- second holds and add 5 seconds each week. Perform 3 reps each week.

Cardio
15-30 minutes on any piece of cardiovascular equipment using steady-state effort. This is a pace where you could just about hold a breathless conversation.
Perform this after your resistance training, twice a week.

Workouts
3 each week.

Week 1
a) 2 x 10 reps
b) 2 x 12 reps
c) 2 x 14 reps

Week 2
a) 3 x 10 reps
b) 3 x 10 reps
c) 3 x 10 reps

Week 3
a) 3 x 12 reps
b) 3 x 12 reps
c) 3 x 14 reps

Week 4
a) 3 x 16 reps
b) 3 x 17 reps
c) 3 x 18 reps

Speed of lift
1:2

Rest
2 minutes between sets and exercises.

MONTH 1 workout

1 Bench triceps dip
Targets: triceps

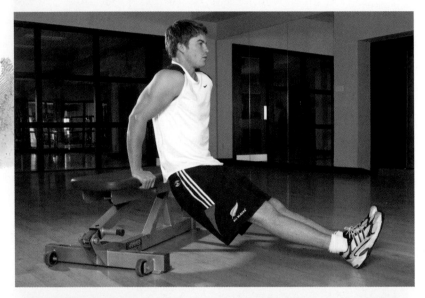

- Grip the bench with your hands facing forward.
- Look straight ahead.
- Keep your legs straight.

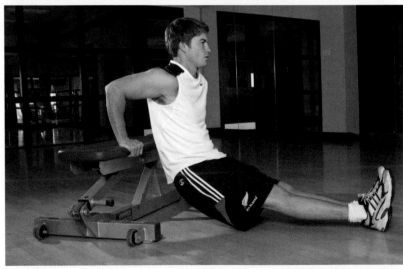

- Resist the temptation to use your legs to lift your body.
- Use your arms to push back up.

2 Crunch
Targets: abdominals

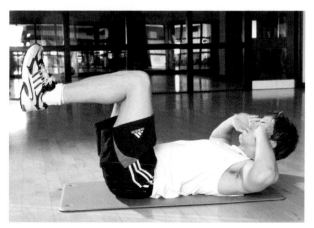 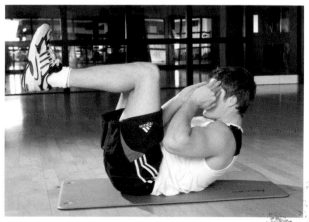

■ Line your elbows up with your ears.
■ Don't hold your head.

■ Focus on contracting your abdominals to lift your torso.
■ Don't lift too high.
■ Lower your body with control.

3 Plank
Targets: core

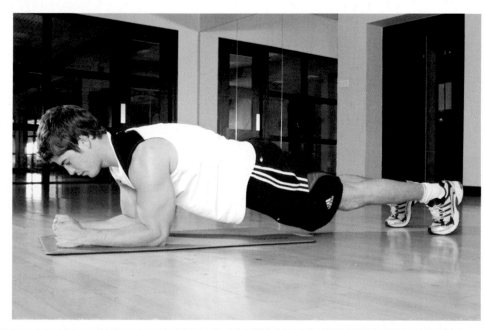

■ Look down.
■ Keep a straight line from head to heels.
■ Place your elbows beneath your shoulders.
■ Relax in the held position.

MONTH 1
workout

 Lunge
Targets: thighs and glutes

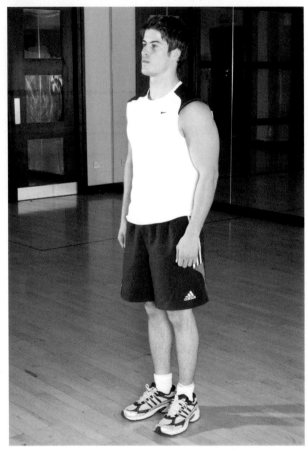 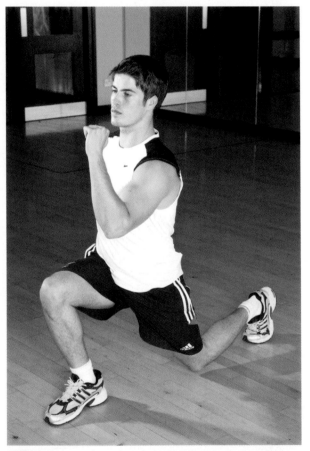

- Stand tall.
- Keep looking forward throughout the exercise.
- Take a large step forward with your right foot.

- Place your right foot flat on the ground, and bend your right leg until your thigh is at right angles to the floor.
- Don't extend your right knee past your toes.
- Keep your chest up.
- Bring your left arm forward.
- Lower your left knee until it almost contacts the ground.
- Power back with your front leg, and repeat with your left leg.

5 ▶ Swiss ball back extension
Targets: back

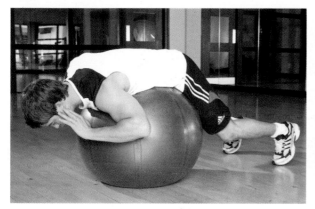

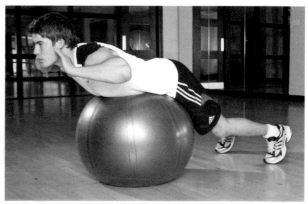

- Place hands by your ears.
- Keep elbows out.
- Maintain hip contact with the ball.

- Don't lift too high.
- Keep hips in contact with the ball.
- Control the lowering phase.

6 ▶ Chest press
Targets: pecs, deltoids and triceps

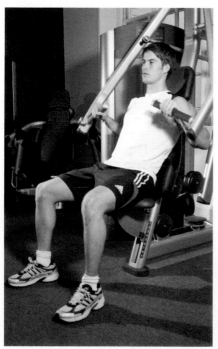

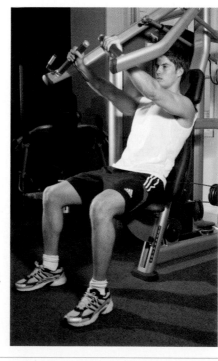

- Brace your core.
- Look straight ahead.
- Maintain natural curve of back.
- Keep both feet flat on the floor.

- Push equally with both arms.
- Control movement on way back.

MONTH 1
workout

7 ▶ Leg press
Targets: thighs and glutes

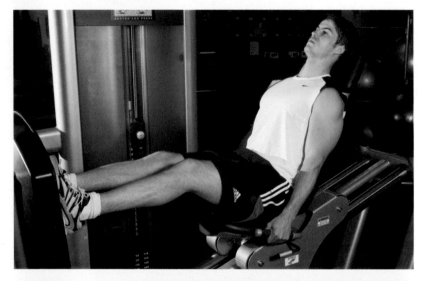

- Look straight ahead.
- Push through both legs equally.
- Extend legs until nearly straight.

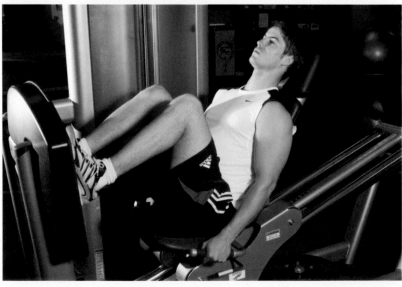

- Control the weights back.
- Stop at a 90° angle at the knee.
- Keep looking forward.

8 ▶ Leg curl
Targets: hamstrings

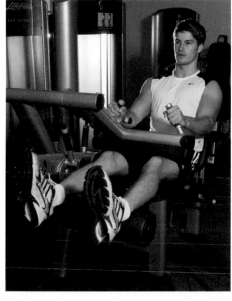

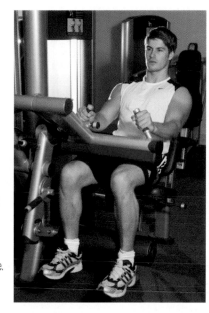

■ Adjust the seat so you are sitting upright or slightly back.
■ Brace your core.
■ Keep looking straight ahead.

■ Pull the pad towards you.
■ Feel the tension in your hamstrings as you return the weights to the start position.

9 ▶ Seated dumb-bell shoulder press
Targets: shoulders

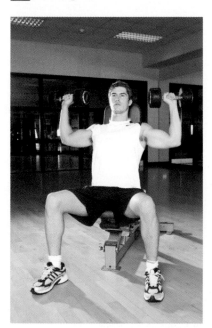

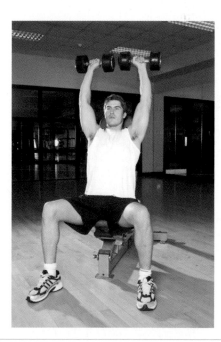

■ Look straight ahead.
■ Hold the dumb-bells at shoulder height.
■ Keep elbows out to the sides.
■ Feet flat on the floor.

■ Don't let the dumb-bells touch at the top of the movement.
■ Ensure core is braced.
■ Maintain natural curves of back.

Meal plan

This high-protein meal plan will give you around 3,000 calories a day

	Monday	Tuesday	Wednesday	Thursday
Breakfast	■ 4 scrambled egg whites on 2 slices of wholemeal toast. ■ 1 grapefruit.	■ Porridge made with 45g oats, 300ml skimmed milk, 1tsp honey and 25g whey protein.	■ 2 slices of French toast made with 1 egg, 1 pint milk, ½tsp cinnamon and ½tsp nutmeg.	■ Porridge made with 45g oats, 300ml skimmed milk, 1tsp honey and 25g whey protein.
Morning snack	■ Mixed nuts, raisins and dried cranberries.	■ 1 mashed banana on 1 slice of wholemeal toast.	■ 120g low-fat yoghurt with blueberries, honey and oats. ■ 1 protein bar.	■ 2tbsp peanut butter. ■ 1 apple. ■ Glass of skimmed milk.
Lunch	■ Turkey and cheese bagel. ■ 1 orange.	■ Turkey-salad sandwich on wholemeal bread. ■ 1 apple.	■ Chicken, bacon and avocado baguette. ■ 1 pear.	■ Medium-sized jacket potato with tuna, baked beans and grated cheese.
Afternoon snack	■ Smoothie: blend 25g whey protein, 80g strawberries, 80g blueberries and 50g blackberries with 200-300ml water.	■ Mixed nuts, raisins and dried cranberries with cottage cheese.	■ Smoothie: blend 25g whey protein 100g strawberries and ½ banana with 300ml skimmed milk and 1tsp flaxseed oil.	■ Smoothie: blend 25g whey protein, 80g raspberries, 80g blueberries and 50g blackberries with 200-300ml water.
Dinner	■ 120g salmon, with stir-fried broccoli, green beans, red peppers and spinach with sesame oil. ■ 70g brown rice.	■ 90g wholemeal pasta and 200g grilled chicken with jar of tomato sauce and chopped onion.	■ 120g tuna steak, with stir-fried broccoli, green beans and spinach with sesame oil and seeds. ■ 70g brown rice.	**Daube of beef**
Bedtime snack	■ Smoothie: blend 25g whey protein, 50g blueberries, 50g blackberries and ½ banana with 300ml skimmed milk.	■ Smoothie: blend 25g protein, 50g blueberries, 50g blackberries and ½ banana with 300ml skimmed milk.	■ 100g cottage cheese and pineapple.	■ 120g low-fat yoghurt with strawberries.
Daily totals	■ 2,857 calories ■ 201g protein ■ 345g carbs ■ 66g fat	■ 2,865 calories ■ 205g protein ■ 363g carbs ■ 64g fat	■ 2,831 calories ■ 200g protein ■ 362g carbs ■ 67g fat	■ 2,945 calories ■ 210g protein ■ 367g carbs ■ 69g fat

Friday	Saturday	Sunday
■ Smoothie: blend 25g whey protein, 100g strawberries and ½ banana with 300ml skimmed milk and 1tsp flaxseed oil. Serve chilled.	■ Porridge, made with 45g oats, 300ml skimmed milk, 1tsp honey and 25g whey protein.	■ 2 scrambled eggs on 2 slices of wholemeal toast. ■ 1 grapefruit. ■ Glass of orange juice.
■ 90g sardines on 2 slices wholemeal toast.	■ 1 mashed banana with 2tbsp peanut butter on 2 slices of wholemeal toast.	■ 30g brazil nuts. ■ Glass of skimmed milk.
■ Medium-sized jacket potato with baked beans and cottage cheese.	■ Turkey, cheese and mustard bagel. ■ 1 apple.	■ Medium-sized jacket potato with baked beans, tuna and grated cheese.
■ 140g grilled chicken, with beetroot.	■ 1 tin of tuna with beetroot. ■ 125g low-fat yoghurt.	■ Smoothie: blend 25g whey protein, 100g strawberries and ½ banana with 300ml skimmed milk and 1tsp flaxseed oil.
■ 200g chicken and vegetable stir-fry with red and green peppers, sesame oil and seeds. ■ 70g brown rice.	■ 120g fillet steak with mashed potato and spinach. ■ Fruit sorbet.	■ 150g roast chicken with 100g new potatoes, and mixed vegetables.
■ Smoothie: blend 25g whey protein, 80g raspberries, 80g blueberries and 50g blackberries, with 200-300ml water.	■ Smoothie: blend 25g whey protein, 80g raspberries, 80g blueberries and 50g blackberries, with 200-300ml water.	■ 100g cottage cheese. ■ 1 apple.
2,869 calories **208g protein** **351g carbs** **63g fat**	**2,950 calories** **210g protein** **359g carbs** **68g fat**	**2,985 calories** **210g protein** **362g carbs** **73g fat**

Daube of beef

serves 2

Ingredients
2 rump steaks
4 strips of streaky bacon chopped
1tbsp plain flour
1tbsp olive oil
8g butter
4 shallots
2 garlic cloves, crushed
500ml beef stock
1 bay leaf,
2 sprigs each of thyme, parsley and marjoram
Salt and black pepper

To make
Preheat the oven to 160°C/325°F/Gas3. Heat a large flameproof casserole dish then add the bacon and cook until golden brown. Cut the beef into cubes, then coat with seasoned flour. Remove bacon from the casserole and put to one side, add the oil and brown the pieces of beef, then set aside. Add the butter to the casserole, cook the shallots and garlic until golden brown. Return the bacon and beef to the casserole and stir in the stock, add herbs. Cover and cook in the oven for 1½ hours or until meat is tender. Season to taste and serve with mashed potatoes and broccoli.

Workout log: month 1

See for sets, reps and times

Theme: Getting ready to train

Date: _____

System: Simple sets, light weights

Speed of lift: 1:2

Rest: 2 minutes between sets and exercises

Exercise	Sets	Reps/Time	Weight
Bench triceps dip			N/A
Crunch			N/A
Plank			N/A
Lunge			N/A
Swiss ball back extension			N/A
Chest press			
Leg press			
Leg curl			
Seated dumb-bell shoulder press			

Cardio record your sessions below

Workout comments:

Self tests (see p36)

Record your performance below to monitor your progress

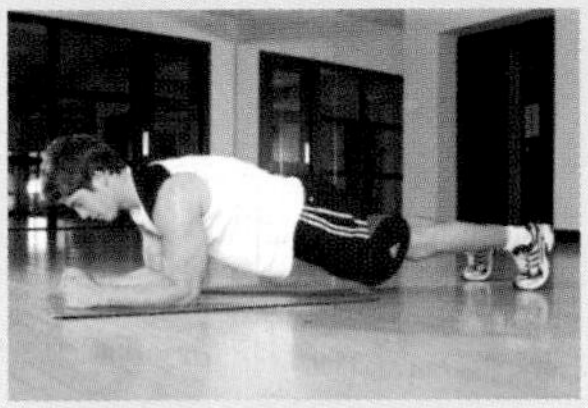

Plank endurance

seconds

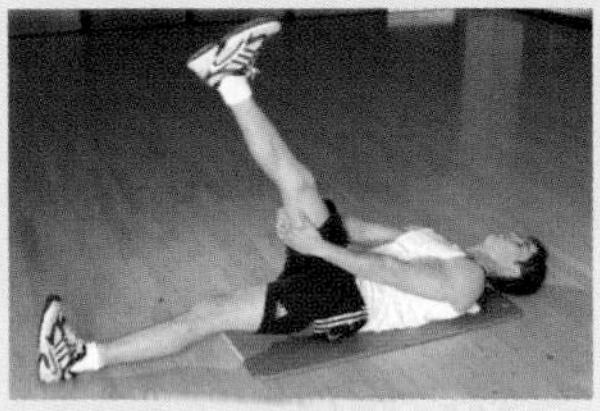

Lying hamstring stretch

seconds

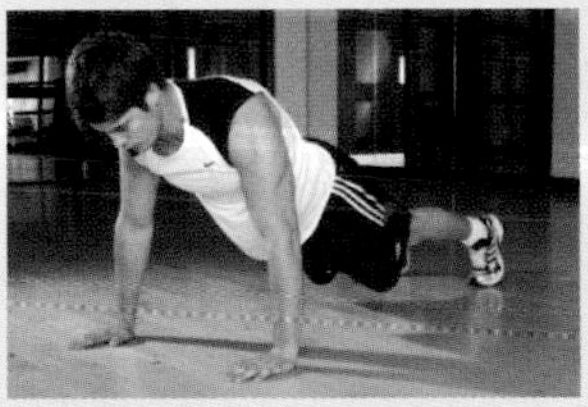

Press-up

number

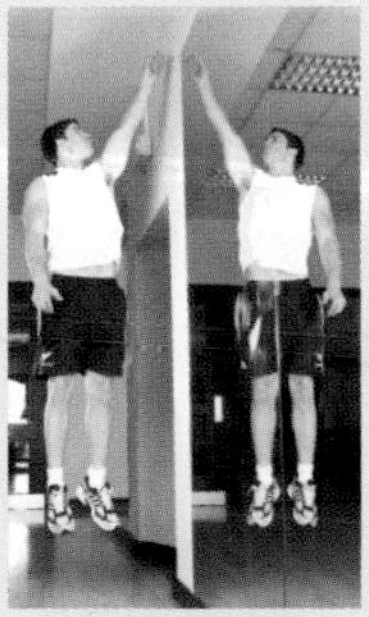

Vertical jump

height

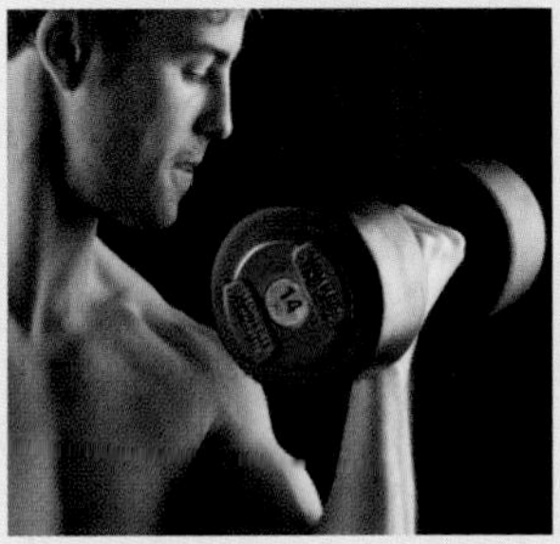

Strength

bench kilograms

squat kilograms

(other)

(other)

Measure up

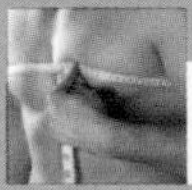

chest

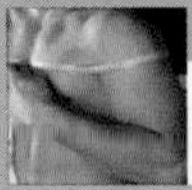

shoulders

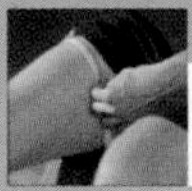

thighs

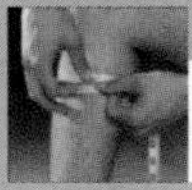

calves

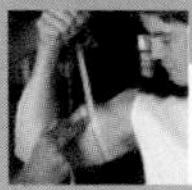

biceps/triceps

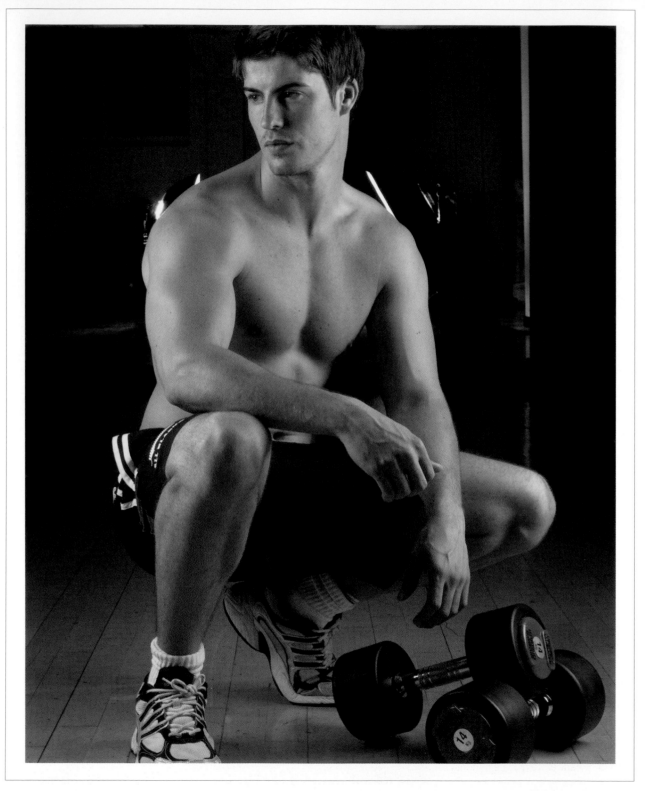

Ultimate Workout Plan

MONTH 2

AIM to handle light-to-medium weights, using simple sets and free weights

AIM to increase cardio fitness so you can recover better between workouts

This month we're going to start to lift some heavier weights, to prepare your muscles for the really heavy stuff to come. Not too heavy though, the weights we'll be using are medium weight. But, even if you think the workouts are too easy, don't be tempted to try and push yourself by moving on to heavier weights too soon. Your body can't continuously adapt on a daily basis. It can only do so optimally in response to a progressive plan that alters loadings

'Don't try to push yourself'

and intensities gradually from month to month. If you were an athlete preparing for the Olympic games, you'd want to feel you were at the peak of your performance as you settled into the starting blocks of the Olympic final. That would mean gradually building up your training over a series of months, a process known as periodisation. The *Ultimate Workout Plan* has been periodised in this way so you'll achieve peak muscle definition by Month 12.

There's an emphasis this month on dumb-bell exercises, this is to stimulate balanced body development. By lifting medium weights, you'll build a great foundation of strength for when you begin to lift heavier weights next month.

Month 2: Getting to know your weights

System
Simple sets, medium weights

Bodyweight
Press-up

Free weights
Dumb-bell bench press
Standing alternate arm dumb-bell shoulder press
Barbell squat
Dumb-bell calf raise

Fixed weights
Leg press
Lat pull down
Leg curl

Core
Plank
Sit-up with twist

For plank, start with 10-second holds and add 2 seconds each week. Perform 3 reps each week.

Cardio
1) 15-30 minute effort as per Month 1.
2) 1 complementary cardiovascular interval training workout (see p28).

Workouts
2-3 each week.

Week 1
a) 3 x 8 reps
b) 3 x 9 reps
c) 3 x 10 reps

Week 2
a) 3 x 10 reps
b) 3 x 11 reps
c) 3 x 12 reps

Week 3
a) 4 x 10 reps
b) 4 x 10 reps

Week 4
a) 4 x 11 reps
b) 4 x 12 reps
c) 4 x 12 reps

Speed of lift
1:2

Rest
2 minutes between sets and exercises.

MONTH 2
workout

Dumb-bell bench press
Targets: pectorals, deltoids and triceps

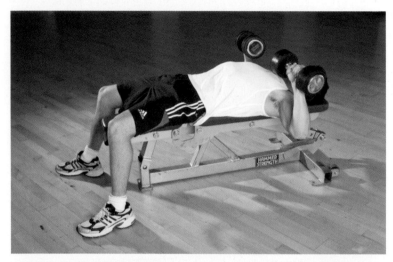

- Support your back and head on bench.
- Maintain the natural curve of your back.
- Hold dumb-bells with thumbs facing each other.
- Hold dumb-bells above chest level.

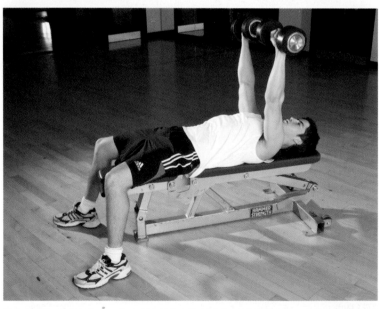

- Press the dumb-bells up over your chest.
- Keep your feet on the floor.
- Don't arch your back.
- Control the movement down.

2 Leg press

Targets: thighs and glutes

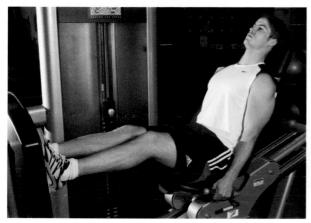

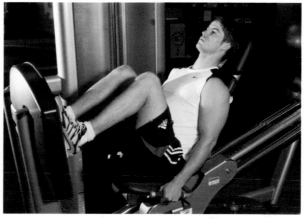

- Look straight ahead.
- Push through both legs equally.
- Extend legs until nearly straight.

- Control the weights back.
- Stop at a 90° angle at the knee.
- Keep looking forward.

3 Standing alternate arm dumb-bell shoulder press

Targets: deltoids

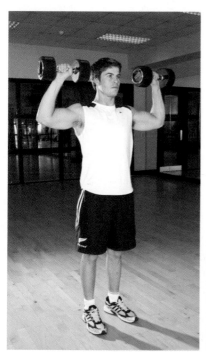

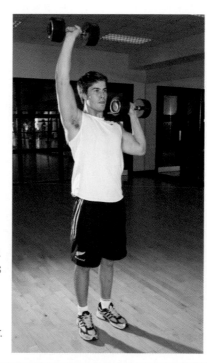

- Look straight ahead.
- Hold the dumb-bells at shoulder height.
- Keep elbows out to the sides.
- Feet flat on the floor.
- Brace your core.

- Press one dumb-bell up over your shoulder at a time.
- Ensure your core is braced.
- Maintain the natural curves of your back.
- Lower under control.
- Alternate sides.

MONTH 2
workout

 Barbell squat
Targets: quads, hamstrings and glutes

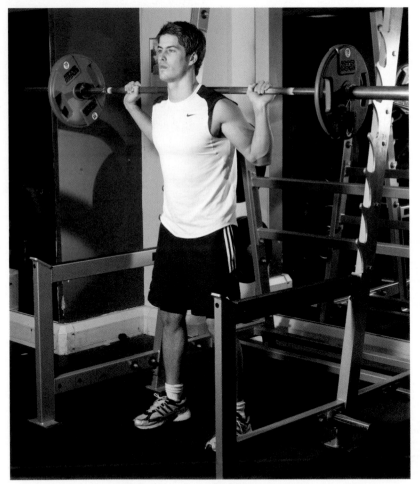

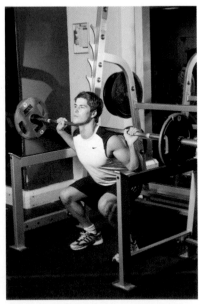

- Take the bar from the rack.
- Rest the bar on the fleshy part of your upper back.
- Look straight ahead and brace your core.

- Maintain the natural curves of your spine.
- Feet shoulder-width apart.

- Lower your torso until your thighs are parallel to the ground.
- Push back through your heels.
- Keep your back naturally rounded.
- Keep looking straight ahead.

5 Dumb-bell calf raise
Targets: calves

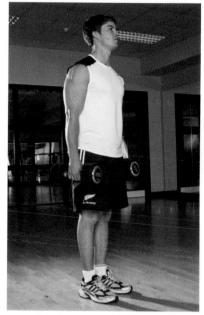

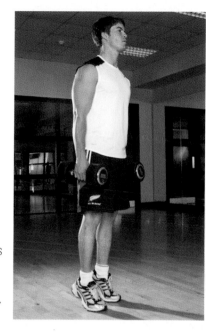

■ Hold the dumb-bells at arms' length by your side.
■ Look straight ahead.
■ Brace your core.

■ Lift your heels off the ground.
■ Keep your toes facing forward.
■ Don't allow your feet to turn in or out.
■ Lower under control.

6 Lat pull down
Targets: lats and upper back

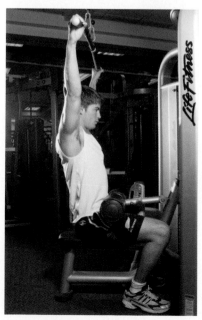

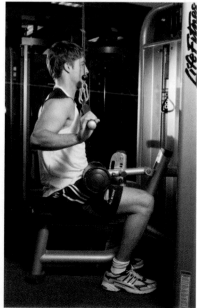

■ Don't lean back too far.
■ Brace your core.

■ Pull the bar to mid chest level.
■ Fix your position and 'feel' your chest work.
■ Feel your lats release and stretch as you return the bar to the start position.
■ Control the movement.

MONTH 2
workout

 7 ## Leg curl
Targets: hamstrings

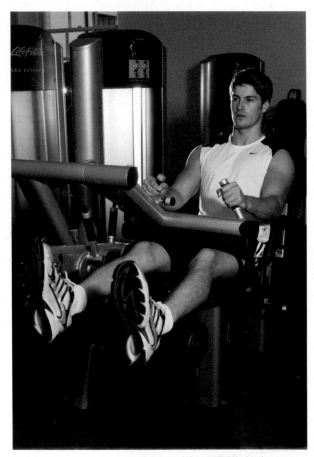

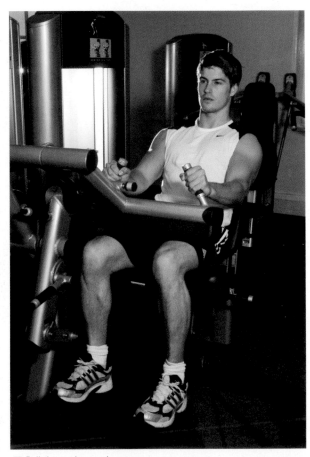

■ Adjust the seat so you are sitting upright or slightly back.

■ Brace your core.

■ Look straight ahead.

■ Pull the pad towards you.

■ Focus on controlling the weight back to the start position, maintaining tension in your hamstrings.

8 ▶ Press-up
Targets: chest, shoulders and triceps

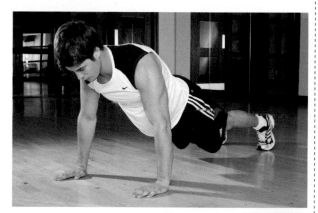

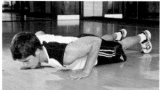

- ■ Keep body in a straight line from head to toe.
- ■ Brace your core.
- ■ Elbows pointing back.
- ■ Lower your body (not your chest).

9 ▶ Plank
Targets: core

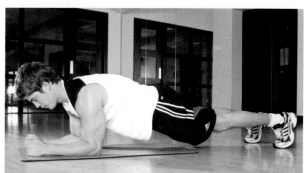

- ■ Look down.
- ■ Keep your head in aligned with your back and legs.
- ■ Place your elbows beneath your shoulders.
- ■ Hold the position.

10 ▶ Sit-up with twist
Targets: abdominals

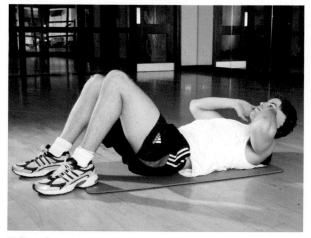

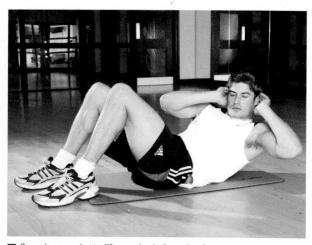

- ■ Place fingers by ears.
- ■ Keep elbows out.

- ■ Crunch your abs to lift your body from the floor.
- ■ Rotate across elbow to one knee.
- ■ Lower under control.
- ■ Repeat to the other side.

Meal plan

This tasty meal plan will help you pack on muscle

	Monday	Tuesday	Wednesday	Thursday
Breakfast	■ 4 scrambled egg whites on 2 slices of wholemeal toast. ■ Glass of orange juice.	■ Porridge made with 45g oats, 300ml skimmed milk, 1tsp honey and 25g whey protein.	■ 4 scrambled egg whites on 2 slices of wholemeal toast. ■ Glass of orange juice.	■ Porridge made with 45g oats, 300ml skimmed milk, 1tsp honey and 25g whey protein.
Morning snack	■ Mixed nuts, raisins and dried cranberries.	■ 1 mashed banana on 1 slice of wholemeal toast.	■ 120g low-fat yoghurt with blueberries, honey and oats. ■ 1 protein bar.	■ 90g mackerel on 2 slices of wholemeal toast. ■ Glass of skimmed milk.
Lunch	■ Turkey and cheese bagel. ■ 1 orange.	■ Turkey salad sandwich on wholemeal bread. ■ 1 orange.	■ Chicken, bacon and avocado baguette. ■ 1 pear.	■ Large jacket potato with tuna, baked beans and grated cheese.
Afternoon snack	■ Smoothie: blend 25g whey protein, 80g raspberries, 80g blueberries and 50g blackberries, with 200-300ml water.	■ Mixed nuts, raisins and dried cranberries with cottage cheese.	■ Smoothie: blend 25g whey protein, 100g strawberries, ½ banana with 300ml skimmed milk and 1tsp flaxseed oil.	■ Smoothie: blend 25g whey protein, 80g raspberries, 80g blueberries and 50g blackberries with water.
Dinner	■ 120g grilled salmon with asparagus and green beans. ■ 70g brown rice.	Jamaican jerk chicken with brown rice	■ 120g tuna steak with stir-fried broccoli, cashew nuts, green beans and spinach with sesame oil. ■ 70g brown rice.	■ 90g wholemeal pasta with 200g grilled chicken, jar of tomato sauce and chopped onion.
Bedtime snack	■ Smoothie: blend 25g whey protein, 50g blueberries, 50g blackberries and ½ banana with 300ml skimmed milk.	■ Smoothie: blend 25g protein, 50g blueberries, 50g blackberries and ½ banana with 300ml skimmed milk.	■ 100g cottage cheese and pineapple.	■ 120g low-fat yoghurt with strawberries.
Daily totals	■ 2,850 calories ■ 199g protein ■ 345g carbs ■ 65g fat	■ 2,919 calories ■ 204g protein ■ 363g carbs ■ 64g fat	■ 2,922 calories ■ 197g protein ■ 365g carbs ■ 69g fat	■ 2,945 calories ■ 205g protein ■ 367g carbs ■ 69g fat

Pre-workout energy smoothie	Friday	Saturday	Sunday
	■ Blend 25g whey protein, 80g raspberries, 80g blueberries, 50g blackberries with 200-300ml water.	■ Smoothie: blend 25g whey protein, 1 mango, 80g blueberries, 2tbsp natural yoghurt and 1tbsp oats with 100ml apple juice and 100ml water.	■ 2 scrambled eggs on 2 slices of wholemeal toast. ■ Glass of orange juice.
	■ 1 mashed banana with 2tbsp peanut butter on 2 slices of wholemeal toast.	■ 90g sardines with lemon juice on 2 slices wholemeal toast.	■ 30g brazil nuts. ■ Glass of skimmed milk.
	■ Turkey, cheese and mustard bagel. ■ 1 apple.	■ Large jacket potato with baked beans and cottage cheese.	■ Large jacket potato with baked beans, tuna and grated cheese.
	■ 1 tin of tuna with beetroot and cottage cheese.	■ 140g grilled chicken with beetroot.	■ Smoothie: blend 25g whey protein, 100g strawberries and ½ banana with 300ml skimmed milk and 1tsp flaxseed oil.
	■ 200g chicken and vegetable stir fry with red and green peppers, cashew nuts, sesame seeds and oil. ■ 70g brown rice.	■ 120g fillet steak with mashed potato and spinach.	■ 150g roast lamb with 100g new potatoes and mixed vegetables.
	■ Smoothie: blend 25g whey protein, 80g raspberries, 80g blueberries and 50g blackberries with 200-300ml water.	■ Smoothie: blend 25g whey protein, 80g raspberries, 80g blueberries and 50g blackberries with 200-300ml water.	■ 100g cottage cheese. ■ 1 pear.
	■ 2,911 calories ■ 194g protein ■ 367g carbs ■ 68g fat	■ 2,943 calories ■ 212g protein ■ 375g carbs ■ 69g fat	■ 3,015 calories ■ 208g protein ■ 367g carbs ■ 74g fat

Jamaican jerk chicken with brown rice

serves 2

Ingredients
200g chicken breasts
1 small onion, chopped
1 small jalapeño pepper, seeded and diced
1tsp ground allspice
1tsp dried thyme
1tsp cayenne pepper
1tsp black pepper
1tsp sage
1tsp nutmeg
1tsp cinnamon
2 cloves crushed garlic
2tbsp soy sauce
1tbsp white wine vinegar

To make
Combine the allspice, thyme, cayenne pepper, black pepper, sage, nutmeg, cinnamon and garlic. Add the soy sauce and vinegar, add the jalapeño pepper, chopped onion and mix. Marinate the chicken breasts in the soy sauce mix for 1 hour. Remove the chicken and baste with the marinade mix. Grill the breasts for 10 minutes on each side or until they are fully cooked and the juices run clear. Serve with brown rice.

Workout log: month 2

See **p53** for sets, reps and times

Theme: Getting to know your weights
System: Simple sets, medium weights
Speed of lift: 1:2
Rest: 2 minutes between sets and exercises

Date: _____

Exercise	Sets	Reps/Time	Weight
Dumb-bell bench press			
Leg press			
Standing alternate arm dumb-bell shoulder press			
Barbell squat			
Dumb-bell calf raise			
Lat pull-down			
Leg curl			
Press-up			N/A
Plank			N/A
Sit-up with twist			N/A

Cardio record your sessions below

Workout comments:

Self tests (see p36)

Record your performance below to monitor your progress

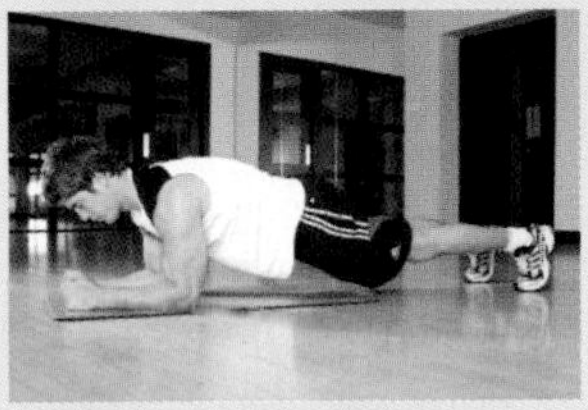

Plank endurance

seconds

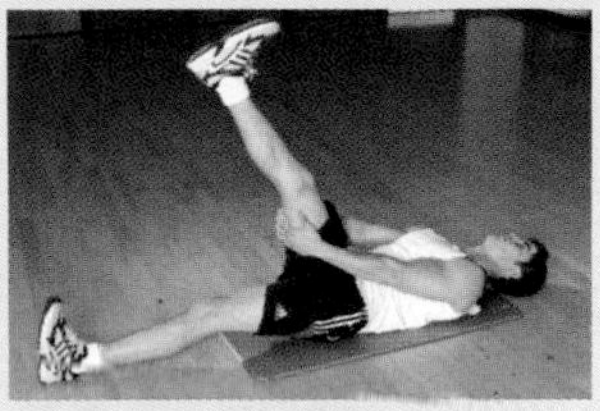

Lying hamstring stretch

seconds

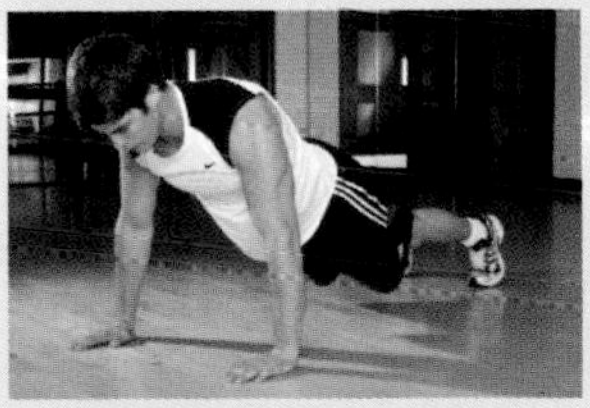

Press-up

number

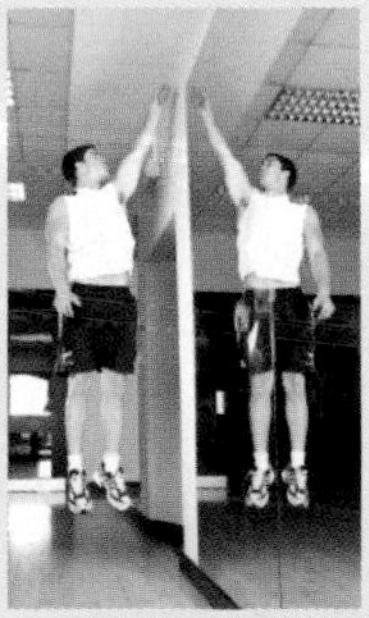

Vertical jump

height

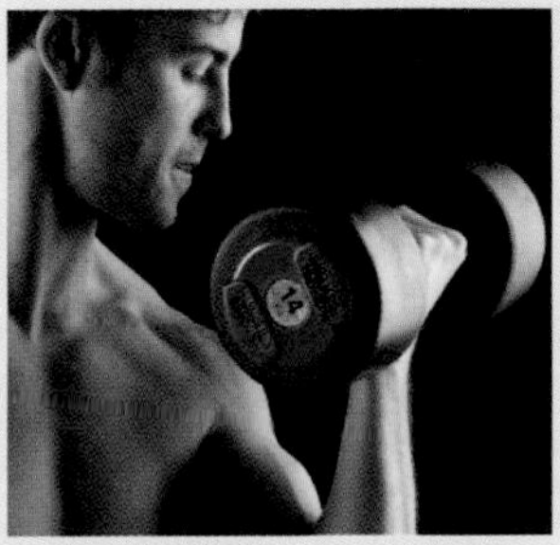

Strength

bench kilograms

squat kilograms

(other)

(other)

Measure up

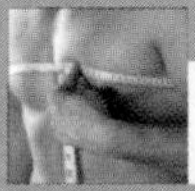

chest

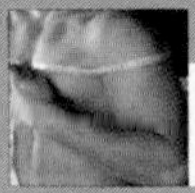

shoulders

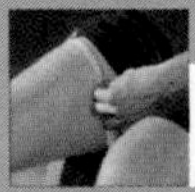

thighs

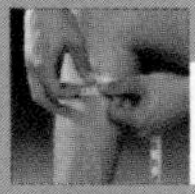

calves

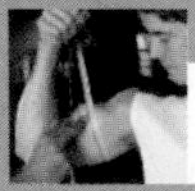

biceps/triceps

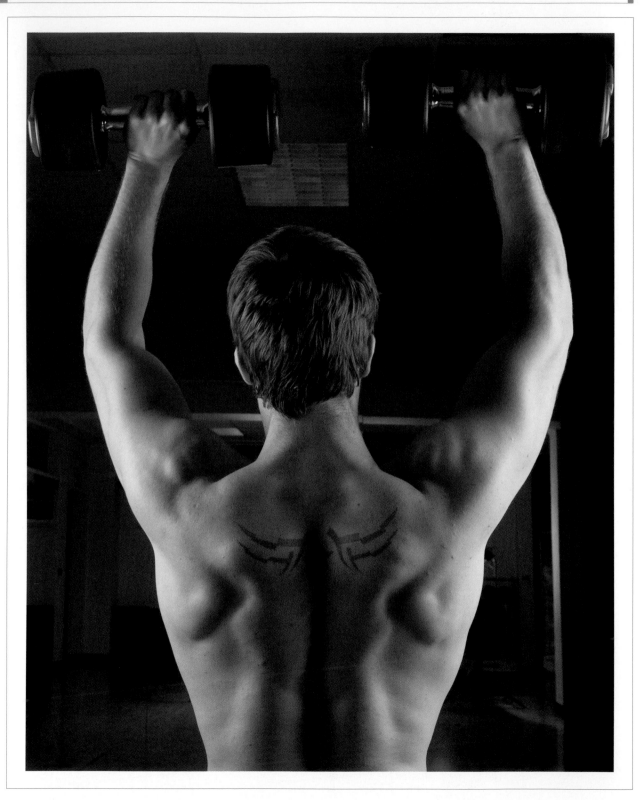

Ultimate Workout Plan
MONTH 3

AIM
to start to build muscle and gain greater strength, using medium and medium-heavy weights

We're ratcheting up the intensity this month. We'll still be using the simple-set system – as a gradual increase in intensity is the aim of the *Ultimate Workout Plan* programme – but there's a much greater emphasis on working to failure. You should be experiencing a degree of difficulty in performing the final reps of each set. If not then you need to increase the weight to push your muscles further.

Repetition variations
compound and isolation exercises + simple sets

Although simple sets generally contain the same number of repetitions for each exercise – for example, 3 x 10 – research suggests that weight trainers of all levels can perform more reps of compound exercises than they can of isolation exercises. So, if you've already increased the weight and you're still able to complete the last couple of reps on the compound moves (moves that work more than one muscle group) without failure, then we suggest that from this month on you add up to four more reps until you achieve failure.

NOTE **Failure must be achieved with good form.**

Month 3:
Lifting heavier – medium-heavy weights

System
Simple sets

Bodyweight
Plank with opposite leg and arm extension

Start with 5-second holds to each side and add 2 seconds each week. Perform 3 reps each side.

Free weights
Barbell front squat
Barbell lunge
Barbell biceps curls
Lying triceps extension using E-Z bar
Standing barbell shoulder press
Barbell bench press

Fixed weights
Seated calf raise
Single-leg press

For the single-leg press, perform the required number of sets for each leg.

Cardio
1) 15-30 minutes effort as per Month 1.
2) 1 complementary cardiovascular interval training workout (see p28)

Workouts

Week 1
a) 3 x 5 light/medium weight
b) 3 x 5 light/medium weight
c) 3 x 6 medium-heavy weight

Week 2
a) 4 x 5 light/medium weight
b) 4 x 5 light/medium weight
c) 4 x 6 medium-heavy weight

Week 3
a) 3 x 12 medium weight
b) 4 x 10 medium weight
c) 4 x 6 medium-heavy weight

Week 4
a) 6 x 4 medium-heavy weight
b) 4 x 10 medium weight
c) 5 x 5 medium-heavy weight

Speed of lift
1:2

Rest
2 minutes between sets and exercises.

MONTH 3
workout

1 Barbell front squat

Targets: thighs and glutes (throws more emphasis onto quads, particularly the outer portion, than back squat)

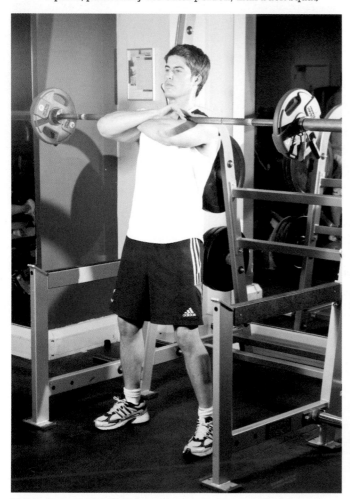

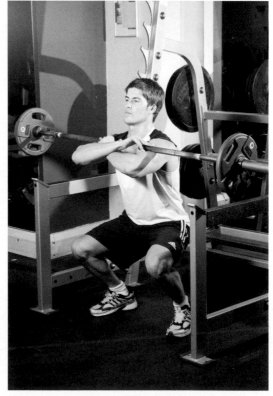

- Take the bar from rack and rest it across the tops of your upper arms.
- Keep your upper arms parallel to the floor and your elbows high.
- Maintain the natural curves of your spine.
- Keep your feet just beyond hip-width apart.

- Lower your torso to a position where your thighs are parallel to the ground.
- Push back up through your heels.
- Keep looking forward throughout the exercise.

2▶ Barbell lunge
Targets: thighs and glutes

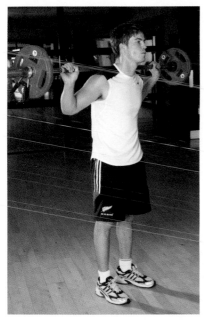

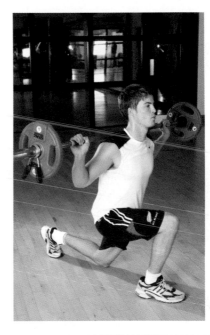

■ Rest bar across the fleshy part of your shoulders.
■ Look forward and brace your core.

■ Take a large step forward.
■ Place your foot flat on the floor.
■ Keep your core braced.
■ Bend your front leg so your thigh is parallel to the ground.
■ Don't extend your knee forward of your toes.
■ Push back up.

3▶ Barbell biceps curls
Targets: biceps

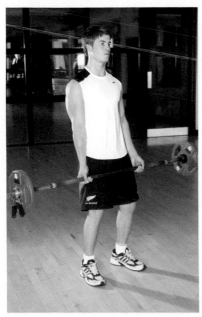

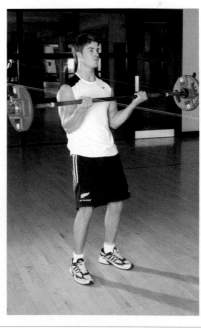

■ Stand tall and look straight ahead.
■ Position your hands just beyond hip-width apart.
■ Keep your elbows in.
■ Brace your core.

■ 'Squeeze' the bar up with your biceps.
■ Lift to a few centimetres from your chest.
■ Lower the bar with control.
■ Keep your elbows pinned to sides.

MONTH 3
workout

4 **Lying triceps extension using E-Z bar**
Targets: triceps

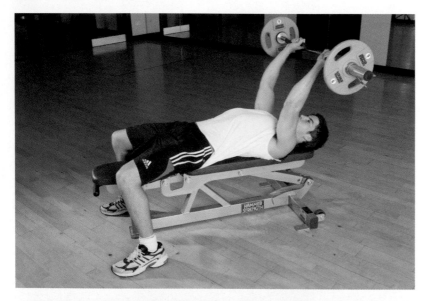

■ Hold the bar over your face
not your chest.
■ Brace your core.
■ Maintain upper body contact
with the bench.
■ Feet flat and in contact with the floor.

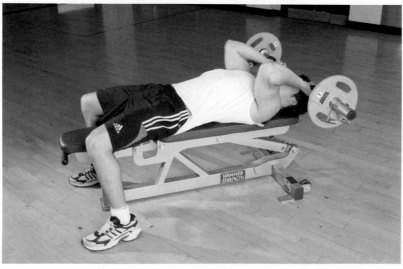

■ Take the weight back.
■ Don't arch back.
■ Keep your upper arms
in the same position throughout.

5 Standing barbell shoulder press
Targets: deltoids

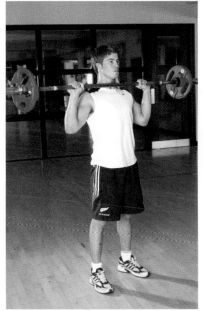

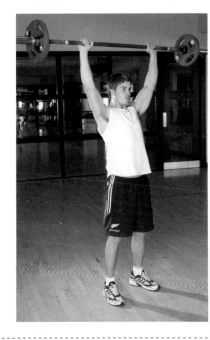

- Brace your core.
- Keep your feet shoulder-width apart.
- Look forward.

- Press bar overhead without leaning backward.
- Lower keeping control of the bar.
- Lower bar to just above upper chest.

6 Barbell bench press
Targets: pecs, deltoids, triceps

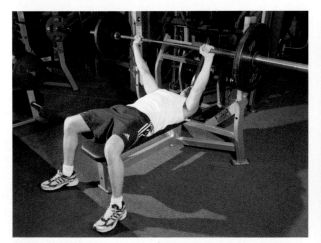

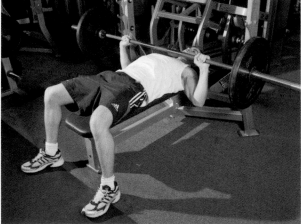

- Take bar from rack.
- Position the bar directly above your chest with your hands wider than shoulder-width apart.
- Maintain natural arch of back.
- Keep your head and shoulders supported on bench.
- Keep feet flat on floor.

- Lower the bar to a centimetre or so above your chest.
- Don't arch your back.
- Keep your feet in contact with floor.
- Press back powerfully.

MONTH 3
workout

7 ▶ Seated calf raise
Targets: calves (soleus)

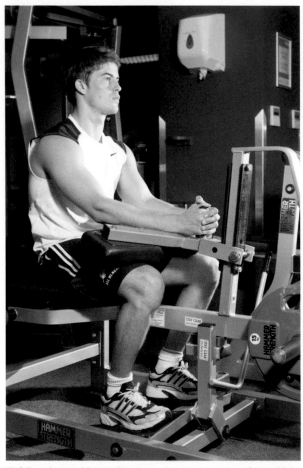 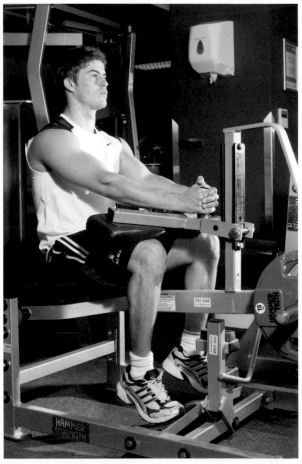

- Adjust the machine so that the pads rest across top of your thighs.
- Look straight ahead.

- Raise your ankles off the ground to lift the weight.
- Control ankles back down.
- Keep your toes facing forward (don't turn your ankles in or out).

8 ▶ Single-leg press
Targets: thighs and glutes

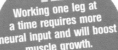

TIP
Working one leg at a time requires more neural input and will boost muscle growth. Be prepared to drop the weight on your weaker side.

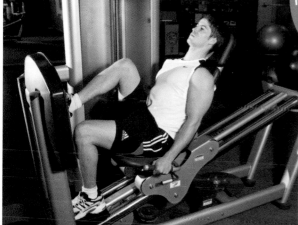

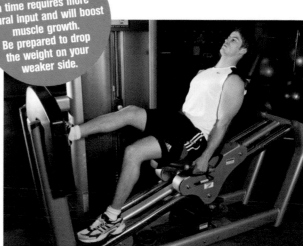

- Look straight ahead.
- Place foot to side of centre line of plate.
- Brace your core.
- Keep leg aligned through hip, knee and ankle.

- Extend the leg until almost straight.
- Control the weight back.

9 ▶ Plank with opposite leg and arm extension
Targets: core

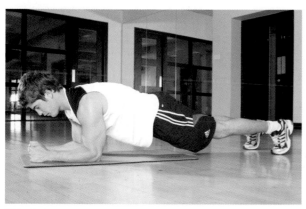

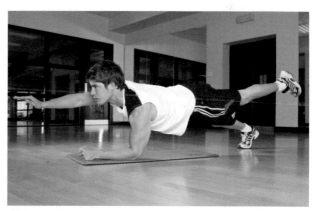

- Look down.
- Maintain balance.
- Pull your abdominals in to create stability.

- Lift opposite arm and leg.
- Lower arm and leg and then repeat with other arm and leg.

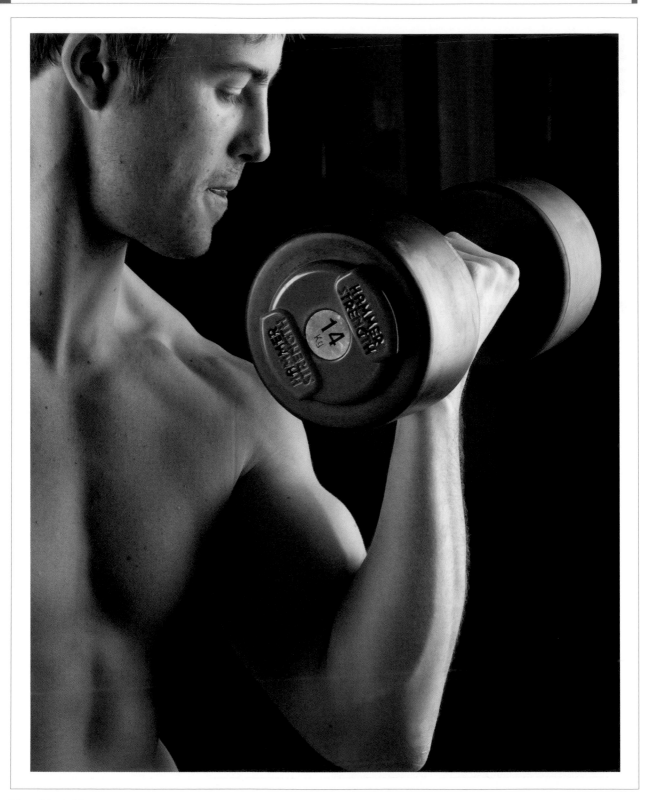

Ultimate Workout Plan
MONTH 4

We're sticking with simple sets this month, but instead of gradually increasing the reps with each workout we're simply increasing the reps week by week. We'll also be using just medium weights rather than the heavy weights of last month. The key difference will be the increase in the speed of the lift from the 1:2

'This increase in speed will have a significant anabolic effect'

method to the 1:1 method. This will have a significant anabolic effect and boost your muscle building hormones. Despite the emphasis on speed, you must maintain good lifting form.

Key muscle building hormone

Testosterone and growth hormone are the key muscle building hormones. Hormones are 'chemical messengers' triggering numberous bodily funtions. The more intense your workout the greater will be the testosterone and growth homone response.

Month 4: Lifting medium weights powerfully

System
Simple sets

Free weights
Barbell front squat
Barbell step-up
Barbell bent-over row
Barbell high pull
Barbell bench press
Barbell calf raise

Fixed weights
Single-leg press

Core
Side plank

Perform 2 reps every other workout session. Holding each side position twice, for as long as you can, with 2-minute recovery between set reps.

Cardio
1) 15-20 minutes effort.
2) 1 complementary cardiovascular interval training workout (see p28).

Workouts

Week 1
a) 3 x 8 medium weight
b) 3 x 8 medium weight
c) 3 x 8 medium weight

Week 2
a) 3 x 10 medium weight
b) 3 x 10 medium weight
c) 3 x 10 medium weight

Week 3
a) 4 x 8 medium weight
b) 4 x 8 medium weight
c) 4 x 8 medium weight

Week 4
a) 4 x 10 medium weight
b) 4 x 10 medium weight
c) 4 x 10 medium weight

Speed of lift
1:1
For barbell calf raise use 1:6

Rest
2 minutes between sets
and exercises

MONTH 4
workout

1 Barbell front squat

Targets: thighs and glutes (throws more emphasis onto quads, particularly the outer portion, than back squat)

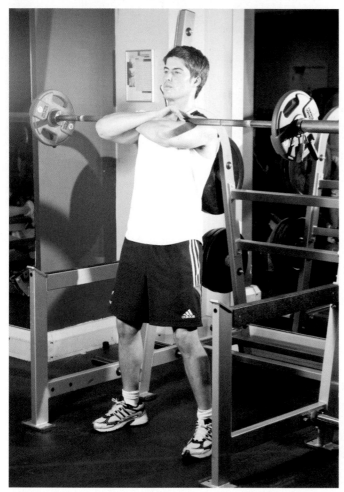

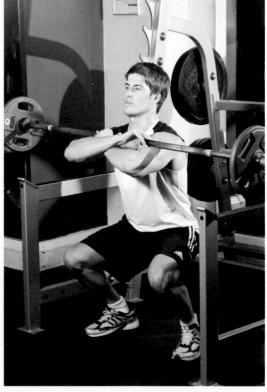

- Take the bar from rack and rest it across the fronts of your shoulders.
- Keep your upper arms parallel to the floor and your elbows high.
- Maintain the natural curves of your spine.
- Keep your feet just beyond hip-width apart.

- Lower your torso to a position where your thighs are parallel to the ground.
- Push back up through your heels.
- Keep looking forward throughout the exercise.

2 Barbell step-up
Targets: thighs and glutes

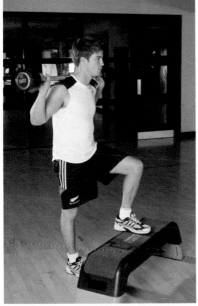

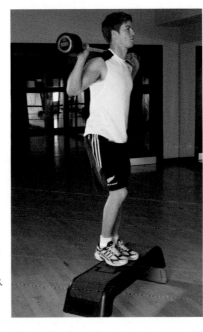

- Look straight ahead.
- Rest bar across the fleshy part of shoulders.
- Place your left foot firmly on the step.

- Push up through your left leg
- Push hips forward.
- Keep back braced.
- Bring right leg up to join the left leg.
- Step back down with your right leg.
- Step up again, this time with your right foot, and then continue to alternate legs.

3 Barbell bent-over row
Targets: upper and lower back

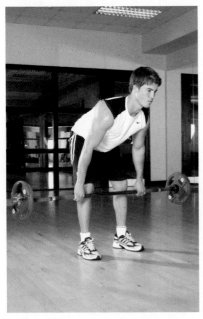

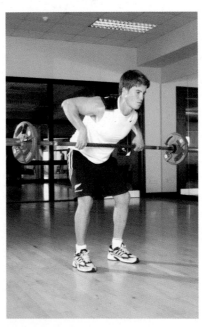

- Keep your feet shoulder-width apart.
- Brace your core.
- 'Hang' the bar around knee height.
- Keep your neck in line with your spine.
- Retract your shoulder blades.
- Maintain the natural curves of your spine.

- Lean from the hips.
- Keep knees 'soft'.
- Hold trunk still.
- Row bar to sternum.
- Control the bar away from you.

MONTH 4
workout

4 **Barbell high pull**
Targets: calves, thighs, glutes, back, shoulders

TIP
This is a really dynamic lift that will significantly boost your muscle-building hormones. Spend some time working out with a light bar before you lift heavier weights.

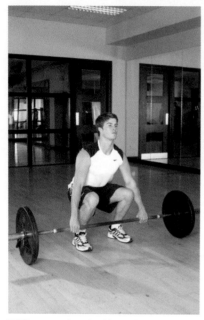

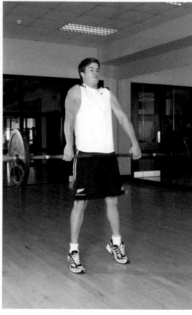

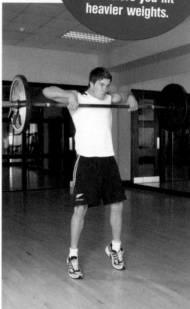

■ Place your feet shoulder-width apart.
■ Hold the bar with your hands slightly wider than shoulder-width apart, using an over-grasp grip.
■ Keep your heels on the floor.
■ Lean slightly back.
■ Keep your arms long.

■ Drive up through your legs.
■ When the bar reaches hip level, push your hips towards the bar.
■ Pull the bar up with your arms.
■ Push up on to your toes.

■ Pull bar to shoulder height.
■ Lift chest and keep head up.
■ Control the fall of the weight.
■ Let your heels return to the floor.
■ Pause, reset and start again.

Barbell bench press

Targets: pecs, deltoids and triceps

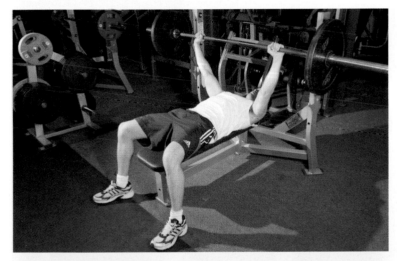

- Brace your core.
- Keep your head and shoulders on the bench.
- Maintain the natural curves of your back.
- Keep both feet on the floor.

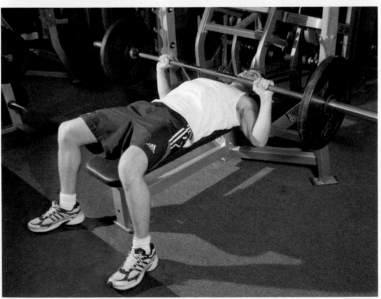

- Lower weights under control.
- Push the weight up powerfully.
- Push evenly with both arms.

MONTH 4
workout

6 ▸ Barbell calf raise
Targets: calves (gastrocnemius)

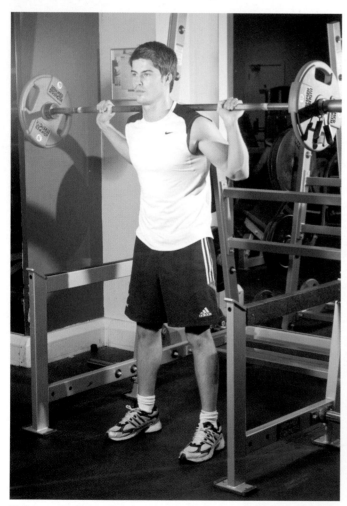

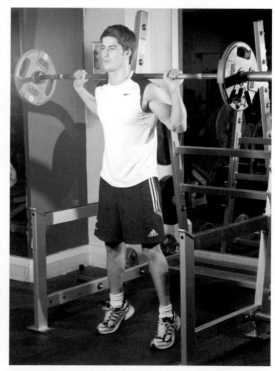

- Remove bar from rack and rest across the fleshy part of your shoulders.
- Keep your head up.
- Brace your abs.
- Place your feet shoulder-width apart.

- Lift your heels off the ground.
- Lower to a count of six.

7 Single-leg press
Targets: thighs and glutes

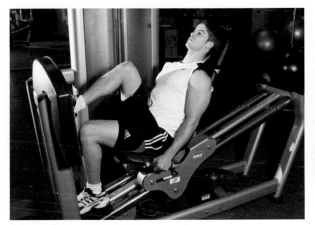

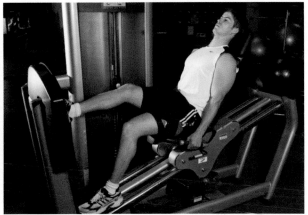

- Look straight ahead.
- Brace your core.
- Place your right foot to right side of centre line of plate.
- Keep your leg aligned through hip, knee and ankle.

- Extend the leg until nearly straight.
- Control the weight back.
- Repeat with your left leg.

8 Side plank
Targets: core

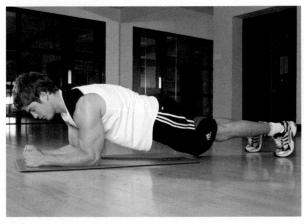

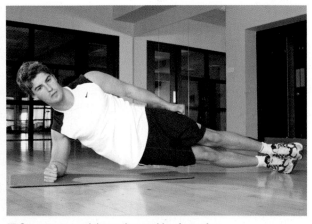

- Get into a plank position.
- Lift and turn your body.

- Support your weight on the outside of your foot.
- Keep your elbow under your shoulder.
- Keep your body in a straight line.
- Keep your upper arm on your side.
- Return to plank position.
- Rotate body and perform to other side.

Meal plan

Fuel your workouts with this muscle-building plan

	Monday	Tuesday	Wednesday	Thursday
Breakfast	■ 4 scrambled egg whites on 2 slices of wholemeal toast. ■ 1 grapefruit.	■ Porridge made with 45g oats, 300ml skimmed milk, 1tsp of honey and 25g whey protein.	■ 2 slices of French toast made with 1 egg, 570ml milk and ½tsp cinnamon and ½tsp nutmeg.	■ 2 scrambled eggs on 2 slices of wholemeal toast. ■ Glass of orange juice.
Morning snack	■ Mixed nuts, raisins and dried cranberries.	■ 1 apple with 2tbsp peanut butter and glass of skimmed milk.	■ 120g low-fat yoghurt with blueberries, honey and oats. ■ 1 protein bar.	■ 1 mashed banana on 1 piece of wholemeal toast. ■ 1 protein bar.
Lunch	■ Turkey and cheese salad sandwich on wholemeal bread. ■ 1 pear.	■ Medium-sized jacket potato with tuna, baked beans and grated cheese.	■ Turkey and cranberry wholemeal sandwich. ■ 1 pear.	■ Turkey salad sandwich on wholemeal bread. ■ 1 apple.
Afternoon snack	■ Smoothie: blend 25g whey protein, 80g raspberries, 80g blueberries and 50g blackberries with water.	■ Smoothie: blend 25g whey protein, 80g raspberries, 80g blueberries and 50g blackberries with 200-300ml water.	■ Smoothie: blend 25g whey protein, 100g strawberries and ½ banana with 300ml skimmed milk and 1tsp flaxseed oil.	■ Mixed nuts, raisins and dried cranberries with cottage cheese.
Dinner	■ 200g chicken and vegetable stir fry with red and green peppers, sesame oil and seeds. ■ 70g brown rice.	Salmon fish cakes	■ 150g lean minced beef chilli with red kidney beans and brown rice.	■ 90g wholemeal pasta and 200g grilled chicken with jar of tomato sauce and chopped onion.
Bedtime snack	■ Smoothie: blend 25g whey protein, 50g blueberries, 50g blackberries and ½ banana with 300ml skimmed milk.	■ 120g low-fat yoghurt with strawberries.	■ 100g cottage cheese and pineapple.	■ Smoothie: blend 25g protein, 50g blueberries, 50g blackberries and ½ banana with 300ml skimmed milk.
Daily totals	■ 2,847 calories ■ 207g protein ■ 345g carbs ■ 65g fat	■ 2,876 calories ■ 201g protein ■ 365g carbs ■ 68g fat	■ 2,837 calories ■ 208g protein ■ 372g carbs ■ 67g fat	■ 2,835 calories ■ 211g protein ■ 362g carbs ■ 62g fat

Friday	Saturday	Sunday
Breakfast smoothie ■ Blend 1 mango, 80g blueberries, 2tbsp natural yoghurt, 1tbsp oats and 25g whey protein with 100ml apple juice and 100ml water.	■ Porridge made with 45g oats, 300ml skimmed milk, 1tsp of honey and 25g whey protein.	■ 2 scrambled eggs on 2 slices of wholemeal toast. ■ 1 grapefruit. ■ Glass of orange juice.
■ 90g sardines on 2 slices wholemeal toast.	■ 1 mashed banana with 2tbsp peanut butter on 2 slices of wholemeal toast.	■ 30g brazil nuts. ■ Glass of skimmed milk.
■ Medium-sized jacket potato with baked beans and cottage cheese.	■ Turkey, cheese and mustard bagel. ■ 1 apple.	■ Medium-sized jacket potato with baked beans and cottage cheese.
■ 140g grilled chicken with beetroot.	■ 1 tin of tuna with beetroot. ■ 1 low-fat yoghurt.	■ Smoothie: blend 25g whey protein, 80g raspberries, 80g blueberries and 50g blackberries with water.
■ 120g tuna steak with stir-fried broccoli, green beans and spinach with sesame oil and seeds. ■ 70g brown rice.	■ 120g fillet steak with mashed potato and spinach. ■ Slice of cheesecake.	■ 150g roast pork with 100g new potatoes, and mixed vegetables.
■ Smoothie: blend 25g whey protein, 80g raspberries, 80g blueberries and 50g blackberries with 200-300ml water.	■ Smoothie: blend 25g whey protein, 80g raspberries, 80g blueberries and 50g blackberries with 200-300ml water.	■ Smoothie: blend 25g whey protein, 100g strawberries and ½ banana with 1tsp flaxseed oil and 300ml skimmed milk.
■ 2,910 calories ■ 212g protein ■ 361g carbs ■ 63g fat	■ 2,985 calories ■ 209g protein ■ 369g carbs ■ 74g fat	■ 2,995 calories ■ 211g protein ■ 364g carbs ■ 71g fat

Salmon fish cakes

serves 2

Ingredients
2 salmon fillets
1 egg white
1tsp chopped fresh parsley
1tsp white wine vinegar
1tsp Worcestershire sauce
½tsp chilli flakes

To make
Beat the egg white in a bowl until thick. In another bowl, combine ground salmon, parsley, vinegar, Worcestershire sauce and red pepper flakes. Then fold the egg whites into the salmon mixture. Spoon the mixture into four salmon cakes and add to an oiled frying pan. Cook over medium heat for 6 minutes, turning occasionally. Serve with brown rice and green vegetables.

Workout log: month 4

See p77 for sets, reps and times

Theme: Lifting medium weights powerfully
System: Simple sets
Speed of lift: 1:1 (except calf raise 1:5)
Recovery: 2 minutes between sets and exercises

Date: _____

Exercise	Sets	Reps/Time	Weight
Barbell front squat			
Barbell step-up			
Barbell bent-over row			
Barbell high pull			
Barbell bench press			
Barbell calf raise			
Single-leg press			
Side plank			N/A

Cardio record your sessions below

Workout comments:

Self tests (see p36)

Record your performance below to monitor your progress

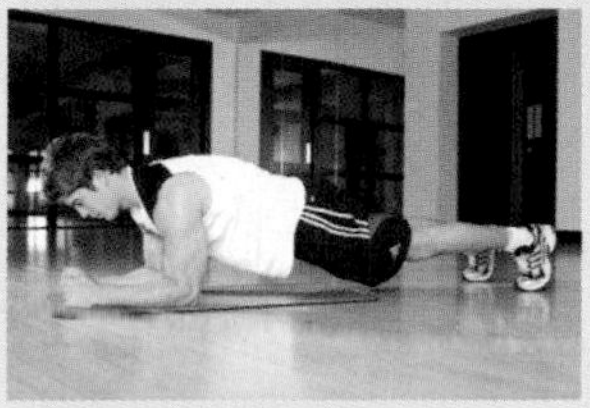

Plank endurance

seconds

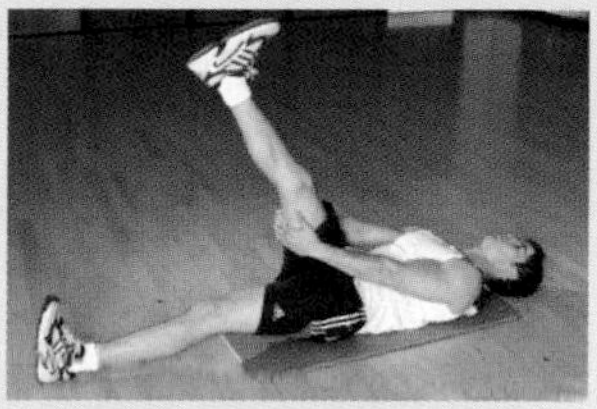

Lying hamstring stretch

seconds

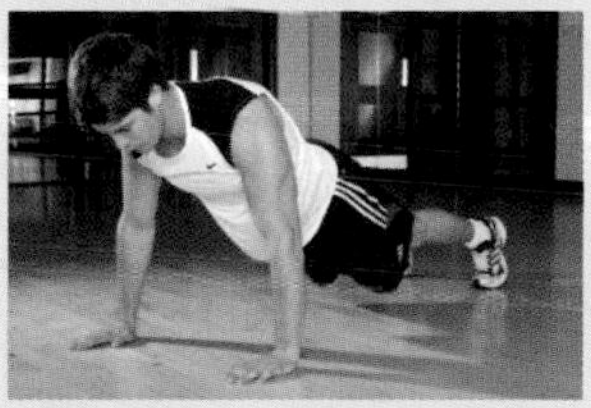

Press-up

number

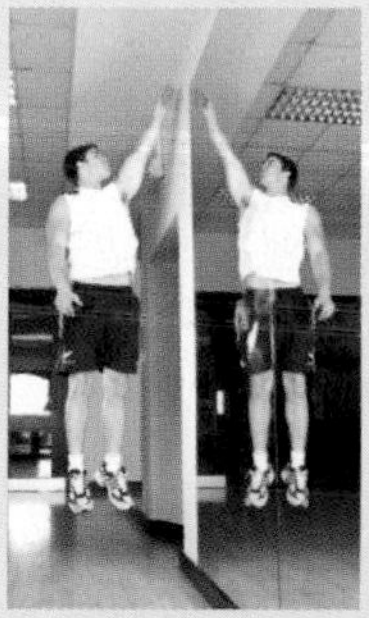

Vertical jump

height

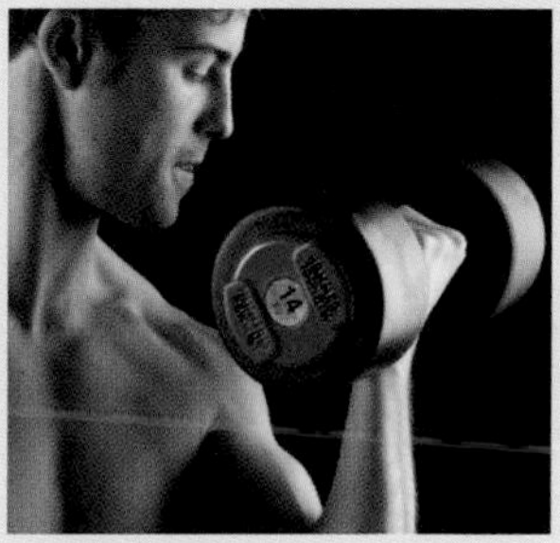

Strength

bench kilograms

squat kilograms

(other)

(other)

Measure up

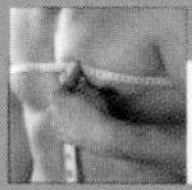

chest

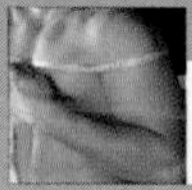

shoulders

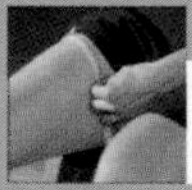

thighs

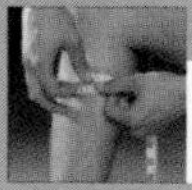

calves

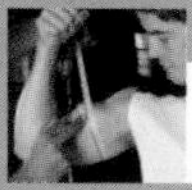

biceps/triceps

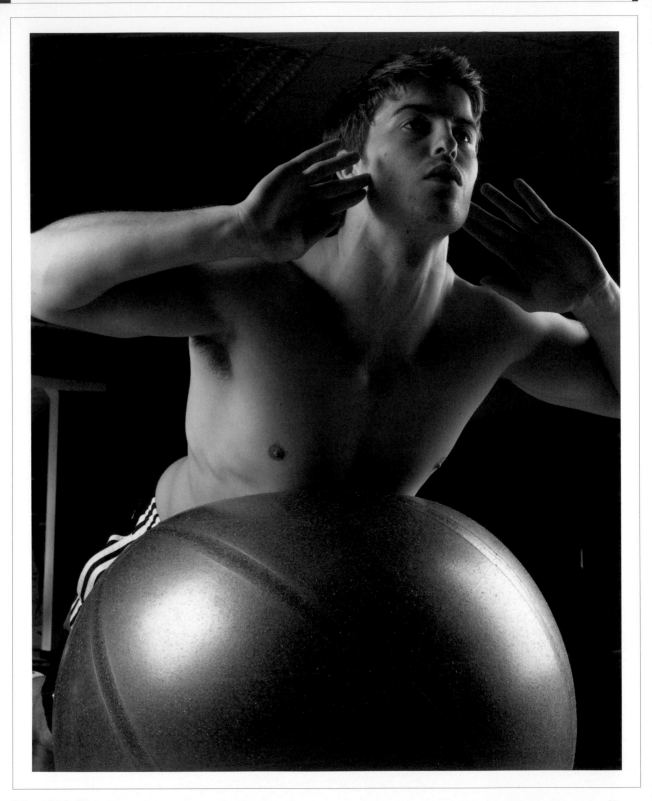

Ultimate Workout Plan
MONTH 5

AIM
to lift heavy weights, using low repetition pyramids and split routine

By now you'll be familiar with most of the key lifts that form the *Ultimate Workout Plan,* and should be up to handling intense workouts. So we'll progress to lifting heavy weights more consistently – ones that will make it difficult for

'As with the power sessions in month four you'll need to be in the zone to complete these workouts'

you to complete the fourth or fifth rep. As with the power sessions in month four you'll need to be in the zone to complete these workouts. You'll need to fire up as many fast-twitch fibres as you can to get the most from your workouts.

We're using the pyramid system for most of the lifts. With this system you start with one set of six reps, then one set of four and finish off with two sets of three, adding more weight for each set. With this you should progress to lifting around 90 per cent of what you could lift on one attempt over the final two sets of three. We've also introduced a split routine where you train different body parts on different days. This maximises muscle growth because you create longer recovery periods before training that body part again.

Month 5:
Strength weights, going heavy

System
Pyramid, split routine
(unless otherwise indicated):
1 x 6, 1 x 4, 2 x 3
Simple sets on selected exercises

Split 1 – legs
Barbell squat
Barbell calf raise
Machine leg curl

Split 2 – chest
Barbell bench press
Dumb-bell flye
Press-up

Split 3 – back/arms
Dumb-bell lateral lift
Barbell deadlift
Lying triceps extension using
E-Z bar

Core
Swiss ball back extension
Crunch

Cardio
2 complementary cardiovascular interval training workouts
(see p28).

Workouts

Weeks 1-4
Perform a different split routine each workout and one core exercise:

Legs
Pyramid system

Chest
Pyramid system, except for dumb-bell flye. For these perform simple sets:
4 x 8 medium weight

Back/arms
Pyramid system, except for dumb-bell lateral lifts and lying triceps extension using E-Z bar For these perform simple sets:
4 x 8

Speed of lift
1:2 (for barbell calf raise use 1:6)

Rest
3 minutes between sets.

Core
Swiss ball back extension and crunch: 4 x 15 reps.

Recovery
1 minute recovery between sets.

MONTH 5
split 1 – legs

1 Barbell squat
Targets: thigh and glutes

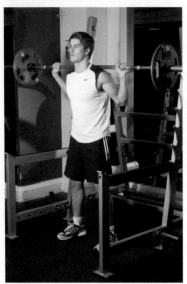

■ Take the bar from the rack and rest it across the fleshy part of your shoulders.
■ Maintain the natural curves of your spine.
■ Keep your feet just beyond hip-width apart.
■ Keep looking forward.

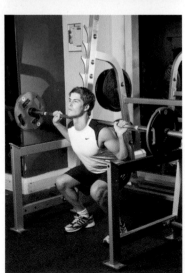

■ Lower your torso until your thighs are parallel to the ground.
■ Push back up through your heels.
■ Keep looking forward.

2 Barbell calf raise
Targets: calf muscles

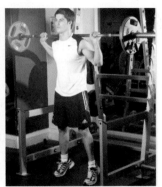
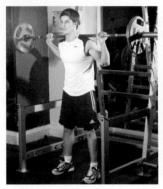

■ Remove bar from rack.
■ Rest it across fleshy part of your shoulders.
■ Keep your head up.

■ Look forward and brace abs.
■ Feet shoulder-width apart.
■ Extend your ankles.
■ Lower to a count of six.

3 Leg curl
Targets: hamstrings

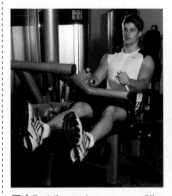
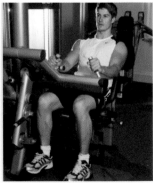

■ Adjust the seat so you are sitting upright or slightly back.
■ Brace your core.

■ Look straight ahead.
■ Pull pad towards you, and feel the tension in your hamstrings.

split 2 – chest

1 Dumb-bell flyes

Targets: chest (reduces the contribution shoulders can make to exercise)

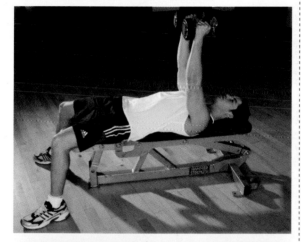

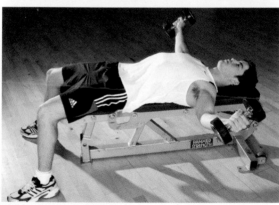

- Hold the dumb-bells, palms facing, directly above chest.
- Support head and shoulders on bench, keep feet on the floor.
- Maintain the natural curves of your spine.
- Take the dumb-bells in an arc out to both sides.
- Lower until the dumb-bells are in line with your shoulders.
- Focus on pecs as you 'pull' the dumb-bells back to the start.
- Don't arch your back.

2 Barbell bench press

Targets: pecs, deltoids and triceps

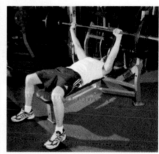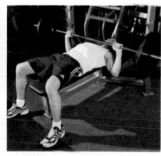

- Brace your core and keep your head and shoulders on the bench.
- Maintain the natural curves of your back.

- Keep both feet on the floor.
- Lower weights under control.
- Push weight up powerfully.
- Push evenly through both arms.

3 Press-ups

Targets: chest, shoulders and triceps

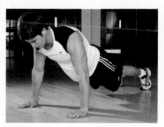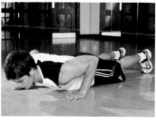

- Keep your body in a straight line from head to toe.
- Brace your core.

- Lower your body, not your chest.

MONTH 5
split 3 – back/arms

1 Barbell deadlift
Targets: back and hamstrings

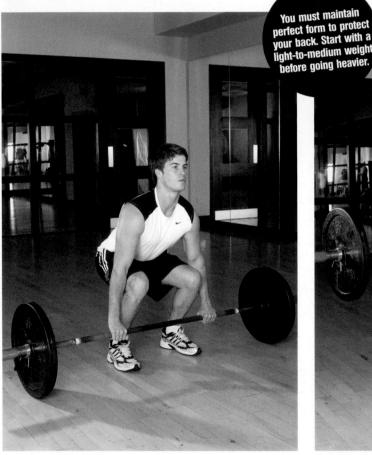

You must maintain perfect form to protect your back. Start with a light-to-medium weight before going heavier.

DEADLIFT Spend the first couple of weeks of this month learning the correct technique before going heavy – practise in your warm-ups.

- Look straight ahead.
- Keep your shoulders back.
- Brace your core.
- Maintain the natural curves of your back.
- Place your feet shoulder-width apart.
- Hold bar with a grip that's slightly wider than hip width.
- Sit back and keep your arms long.

- Push hips forward as you lift bar
- 'Lift' through your bum and back. Don't squat the bar up.
- Keep your neck in line with your spine.
- Keep control on bar as you lower.
- Hold your back in position throughout.

Dumb-bell lateral lift
Targets: side deltoids

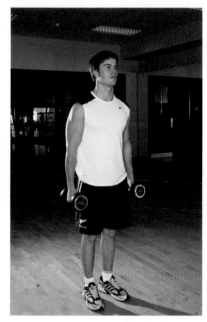

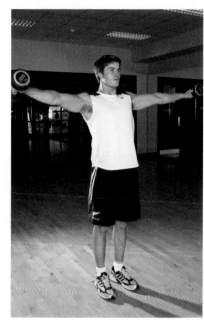

■ Look straight ahead.
■ Maintain the natural curves of your spine.
■ Feet just beyond shoulder-width apart.
■ Hold dumb-bells at arms' length.

■ Lift the dumb-bells to shoulder height.
■ Keep your core braced.
■ Control the weights down.

Lying triceps extension using E-Z bar
Targets: triceps

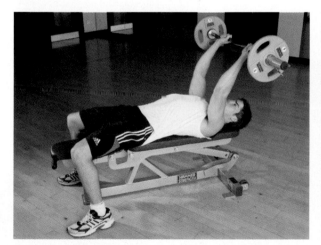

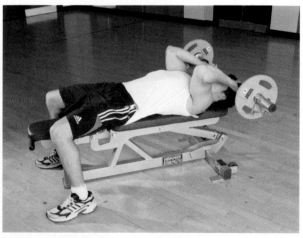

■ Hold the bar over your face, not your chest.
■ Brace your core.
■ Maintain upper body contact with the bench.

■ Fix your shoulders and take the weight back.
■ Don't arch your back.
■ Keep your upper arms in the same position throughout.

MONTH 5
core exercises

1 ## Swiss ball back extension
Targets: back

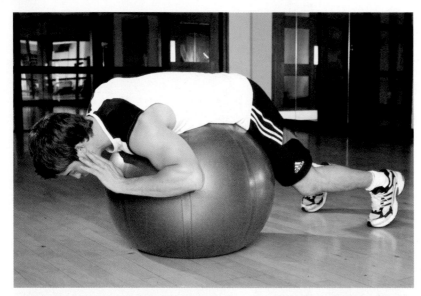

■ Place hands by ears.
■ Keep elbows out.
■ Maintain hip contact with the ball.

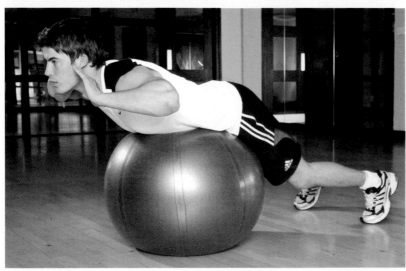

■ Don't lift too high. Keep your hips in contact with the ball.
■ Control the lowering phase.

2 Crunch
Targets: abdominals

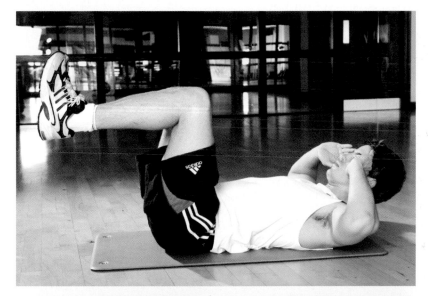

■ Place hands by head, elbows back.
■ Fix your lower legs parallel to ground with thighs at right angles to ground.

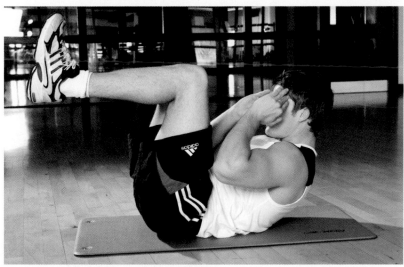

■ Crunch abdominals to lift torso.
■ Lower under control.

Meal plan

Use this 3,000 calories a day meal plan to get the most out of your training

	Monday	Tuesday	Wednesday	Thursday
Breakfast	■ Porridge made with 45g oats, 300ml skimmed milk, 1tsp of honey and 25g whey protein.	■ 4 scrambled egg whites on 2 slices of wholemeal toast. ■ 1 grapefruit.	■ 2 slices of French toast made with 1 egg, 570ml milk, ½tsp cinnamon and ½tsp nutmeg.	■ Porridge made with 45g oats, 300ml skimmed milk, 1tsp of honey and 25g whey protein.
Morning snack	■ 1 mashed banana on 1 slice of wholemeal toast.	■ Mixed nuts, raisins and dried cranberries.	■ 120g low-fat yoghurt with blueberries, honey and oats. ■ 1 protein bar.	■ 1 apple with 2tbsp peanut butter. ■ Glass of skimmed milk.
Lunch	■ Tuna sandwich on wholemeal bread. ■ 1 apple.	■ Turkey and cheese bagel. ■ 1 orange.	■ Chicken, bacon and avocado baguette. ■ 1 pear.	■ Medium-sized jacket potato with tuna, baked beans and grated cheese.
Afternoon snack	■ Mixed nuts, raisins and dried cranberries with cottage cheese.	■ Smoothie: blend 25g whey protein, 80g strawberries, 80g blueberries and 50g blackberries with 200-300ml water.	■ Smoothie: blend 25g whey protein, 100g strawberries and ½ banana with 300ml skimmed milk and 1tsp flaxseed oil.	■ Smoothie: blend 25g whey protein, 80g raspberries, 80g blueberries and 50g blackberries with 200-300ml water.
Dinner	■ 90g wholemeal pasta and 200g grilled chicken with jar of tomato sauce and chopped onion.	■ 120g salmon with stir-fried broccoli, green beans, red peppers, spinach with sesame oil. ■ 70g brown rice.	■ 120g tuna steak with stir-fried broccoli, green beans and spinach with sesame oil and seeds. ■ 70g brown rice.	Chicken Basque
Bedtime snack	■ Smoothie: blend 25g whey protein, 50g blueberries, 50g blackberries and ½ banana with 300ml skimmed milk.	■ Smoothie: blend 25g whey protein, 50g blueberries, 50g blackberries and ½ banana with 300ml skimmed milk.	■ 100g cottage cheese and pineapple.	■ 120g low-fat yoghurt with strawberries.
Daily totals	2,868 calories 196g protein 363g carbs 63g fat	2,857 calories 203g protein 345g carbs 66g fat	2,831 calories 200g protein 362g carbs 67g fat	2,945 calories 210g protein 367g carbs 69g fat

Friday	Saturday	Sunday
■ Porridge made with 45g oats, 300ml skimmed milk, 1tsp of honey and 25g whey protein.	**Muesli smoothie** ■ Blend 1apple, ½ banana, 100g strawberries, 2tbsp yoghurt and handful of muesli with 4 ice cubes.	■ 2 scrambled eggs on 2 slices of wholemeal toast. ■ 1 grapefruit. ■ Glass of orange juice.
■ 1 mashed banana with 2tbsp peanut butter on 2 slices of wholemeal toast.	■ 90g sardines on 2 slices wholemeal toast.	■ 30g brazil nuts. ■ Glass of skimmed milk.
■ Turkey, cheese and mustard bagel. ■ 1 apple.	■ Medium-sized jacket potato with baked beans and cottage cheese.	■ Medium-sized jacket potato with baked beans, tuna and grated cheese.
■ 1 tin of tuna with beetroot. ■ 1 low-fat yoghurt.	■ 140g grilled chicken with beetroot.	■ Smoothie: blend 25g whey protein, 100g strawberries, ½ banana with 300ml skimmed milk and 1tsp flaxseed oil.
■ 120g fillet steak with mashed potato and spinach. ■ Fruit sorbet.	■ 200g chicken and vegetable stir fry with red and green peppers, sesame oil and seeds. ■ 70g brown rice.	■ 150g roast beef with 100g new potatoes, and mixed vegetables.
■ Smoothie: blend 25g whey protein, 80g raspberries, 80g blueberries and 50g blackberries with 200-300ml water.	■ Smoothie: blend 25g whey protein, 80g raspberries, 80g blueberries and 50g blackberries with 200-300ml water.	■ 100g cottage cheese. ■ 1 apple.
2,950 calories **208g protein** **359g carbs** **68g fat**	**2,869 calories** **210g protein** **361g carbs** **63g fat**	**2,985 calories** **210g protein** **362g carbs** **73g fat**

Chicken Basque

serves 2

Ingredients
2 chicken breasts, cubed
1 large onion, chopped,
1 large red pepper, sliced
1tbsp olive oil
2 cloves garlic, crushed
1 tin (400g) tomatoes
1tsp herbs de Provençe
570ml chicken stock
1tbsp plain flour
Salt, pepper and cayenne pepper to season
Parsley to garnish

To make
Fry the onions until light brown, add the garlic and red peppers and fry until softened. Remove onions, garlic and peppers from pan. Fry the chicken on both sides until golden brown. Return the pepper, onion and garlic, to the pan and then slowly mix in the flour and stir in the chicken stock, tomatoes and herbs. Season to taste. Either simmer on the hob on a low heat for 1 hour or transfer to a low oven (150°C/300°F/ Gas2) for 1 hour. Garnish with parsley. Serve with fresh greens and new potatoes.

Workout log: month 5

See p89 for sets, reps and times

Theme: Strength weights, going heavy
System: Pyramid split routine and simple sets
Speed of lift: 1:2 (except calf raise 1:5)
Recovery: 3 minutes between sets and exercises

Date: _____

Exercise	Sets	Reps/Time	Weight
Split 1 – legs			
Barbell squat			
Barbell calf raise			
Leg curl			
Split 2 – chest			
Dumb-bell flye			
Barbell bench press			
Press-up			N/A
Split 3 – back/arms			
Barbell deadlift			
Dumb-bell lateral lift			
Lying triceps extension using E-Z bar			
Core			
Swiss ball back extension			N/A
Crunch			N/A
Plank			N/A

Cardio record your sessions below

Workout comments:

Self tests (see p36)

Record your performance below to monitor your progress

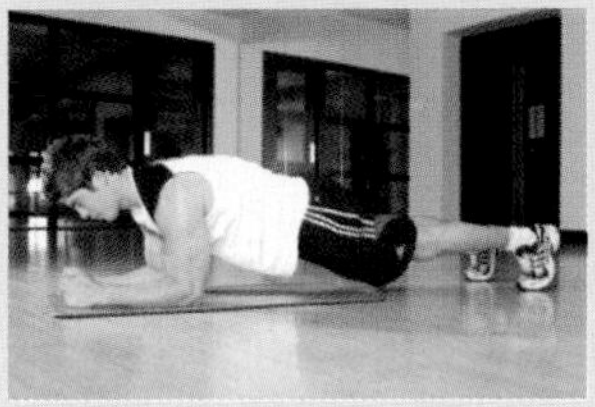

Plank endurance

seconds

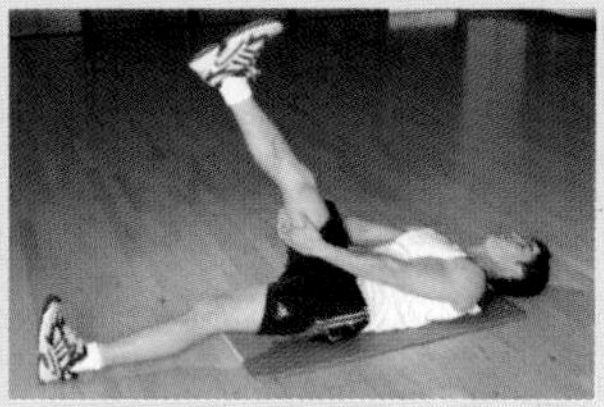

Lying hamstring stretch

seconds

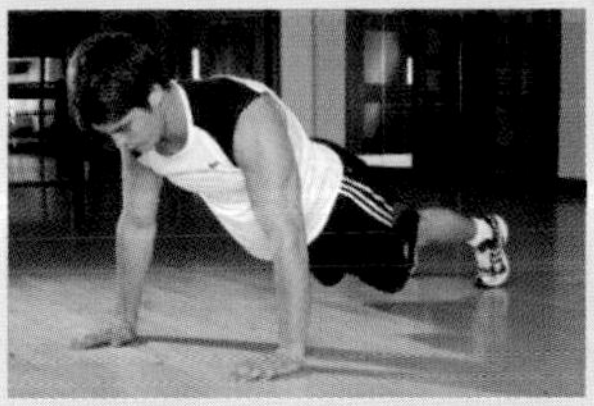

Press-up

number

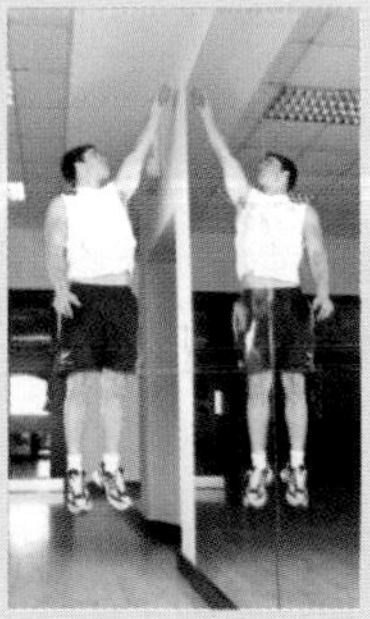

Vertical jump

height

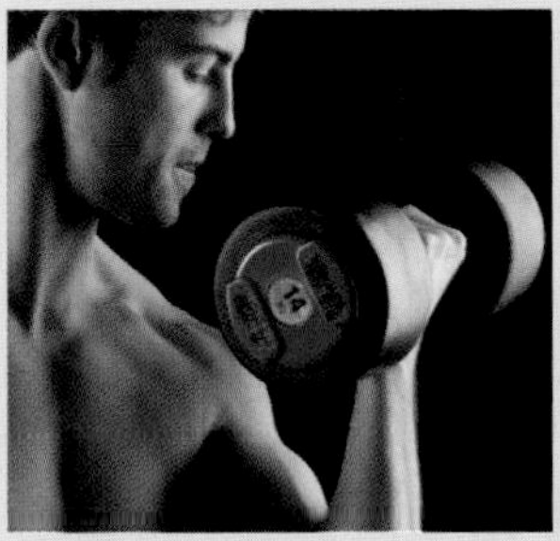

Strength

bench kilograms

squat kilograms

(other)

(other)

Measure up

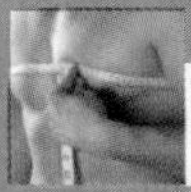

chest

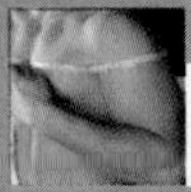

shoulders

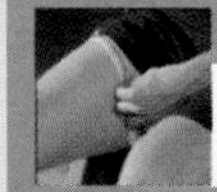

thighs

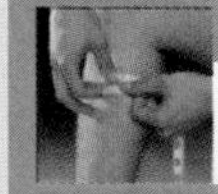

calves

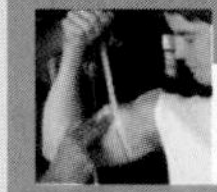

biceps/triceps

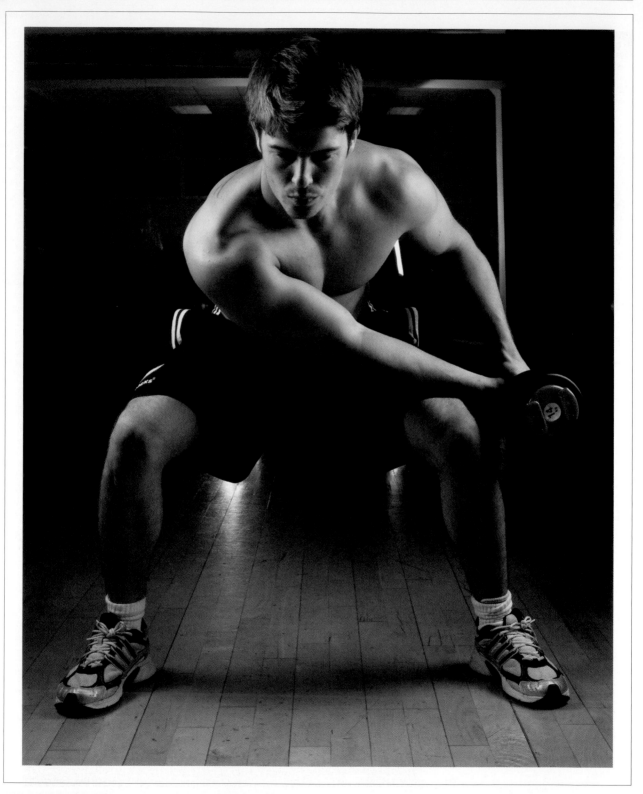

Ultimate Workout Plan
MONTH 6

AIM
to capitalise on the hormonal response of intense weight-training sessions to stimulate muscular growth, using simple sets

Now you've been training for five months it's time to start playing with the big boys. This month we'll be getting a real pump going on, using a typical body-builder's workout that's made up of lots of reps (ten) and sets (four to eight), with minimum recovery (one minute) and using medium weights. There's no getting away form it: this will hurt. But it shouldn't hurt that much. If you recognise any of the signs of over-training (see p15) then you should cut out a workout or train really lightly – you could drop the weight or the number of sets, or both.

The emphasis this month is on building muscle, and so we've cut down the cardio workouts to just one recovery session each week. This should be an easy paced 20-minute effort, which you can do after one of your weights workouts.

Month 6:
High-intensity growth month

System	Workouts
Simple sets	
Lifting medium weights, quickly, with minimum recoveries	**Week 1**
	a) 4 x 10
	b) 5 x 10
Free weights	c) 3 x 10
Barbell squat	
Barbell split squat	**Week 2**
Seated dumb-bell shoulder press	a) 5 x 10
Barbell bench press	b) 4 x 10
	c) 5 x 10
Fixed weights	
Lat pull down	**Week 3**
Leg curl	a) 5 x 10
	b) 4 x 10
Core	c) 6 x 10
Swiss ball jackknife	
4 x 16 reps	**Week 4**
Perform twice a week	a) 5 x 10
	b) 6 x 10
Cardio	
1 x 20 minutes of easy paced effort	**Speed of lift**
	1:1
	Recovery
	1 minute between sets and exercises

'Now you've been training for five months it's time to start playing with the big boys'

MONTH 6
workout

- -

1 Barbell squat
Targets: thigh and glutes

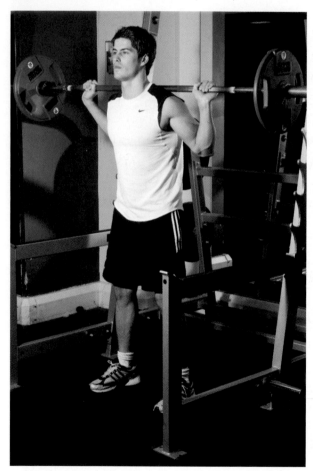
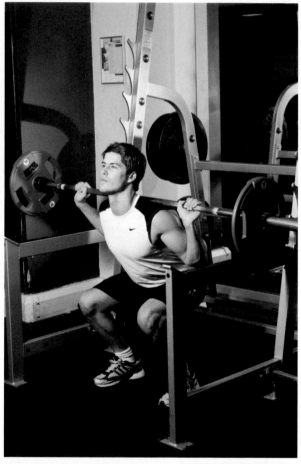

- Take the bar from the rack.
- Rest the bar on the fleshy part of your shoulders.
- Look straight ahead and brace your core.
- Maintain the natural curves of your spine.
- Feet shoulder-width apart.

- Lower your torso until your thighs are parallel to the ground.
- Push back through your heels.
- Keep your back naturally rounded.
- Keep looking straight ahead.

2 Barbell split squat
Targets: thighs and glutes

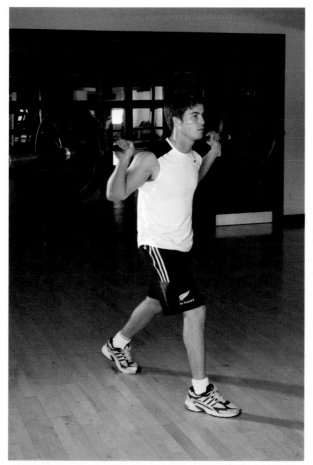

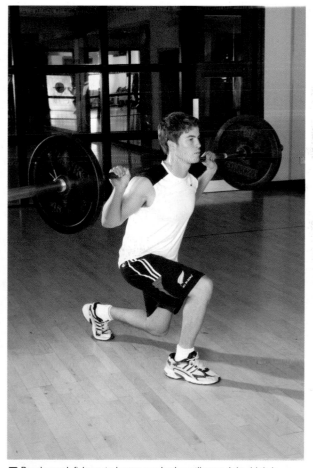

■ Support the bar on the fleshy part of your shoulders.
■ Look straight ahead and take a large step forward
with your right foot.
■ Brace your core and keep your knee behind your toes.
■ Support the weight on the toes of your left foot.
■ Maintain the natural curves of your back.

■ Bend your left knee to lower your body until your right thigh is
parallel to the ground.
■ Think 'bum to floor'.
■ Straighten your left leg to return to the start position.
■ Complete your designated number of repetitions with your right
leg forward and then repeat with your left leg forward.

MONTH 6
workout

3 **Seated dumb-bell shoulder press**
Targets: shoulders

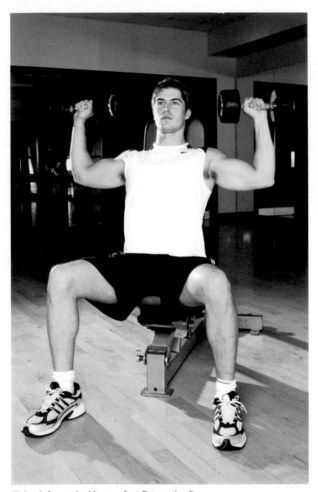

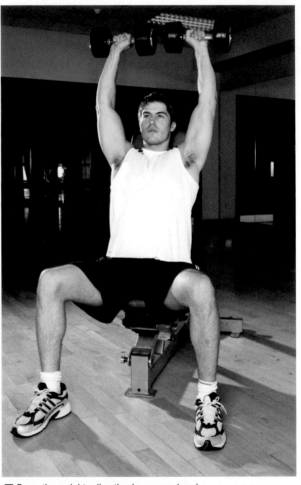

- Look forward with your feet flat on the floor.
- Hold the dumb-bells at shoulder height.
- Maintain the natural curves of your spine with your elbows out to your sides.

- Press the weights directly above your head.
- Don't let the weights touch at the top.
- Keep your core braced.
- Lower the weights under control.

4 **Barbell bench press**
Targets: pecs, deltoids and triceps

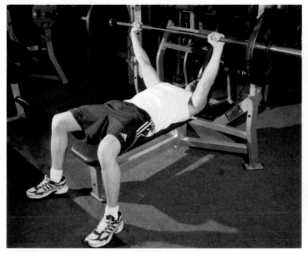 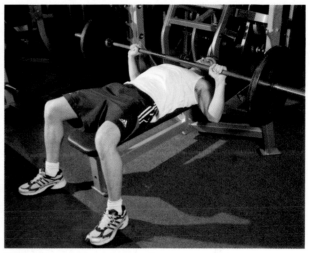

■ Brace your core and keep your head and shoulders on the bench.
■ Maintain the natural curves of your back.
■ Keep your feet on the floor.

■ Lower the weights under control.
■ Push the weight up powerfully.
■ Push evenly through both arms.
■ Do not arch your back as you press.

5 **Lat pull down**
Targets: lats and upper back

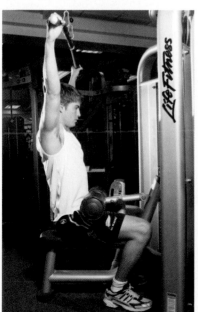 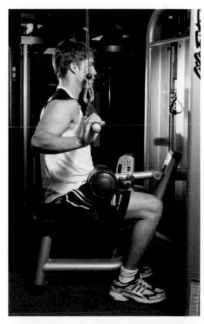

■ Don't lean
back too far.
■ Pull the bar
to mid chest level.
■ Fix your position
and 'feel' your
chest work.
■ Brace your core.

■ Feel your lats
release and stretch
as you return the bar
to the start position.
■ Control the
movement.

MONTH 6
workout

 Leg curl
Targets: hamstrings

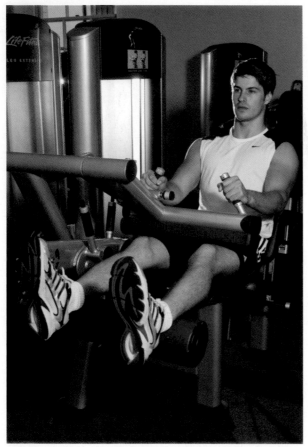 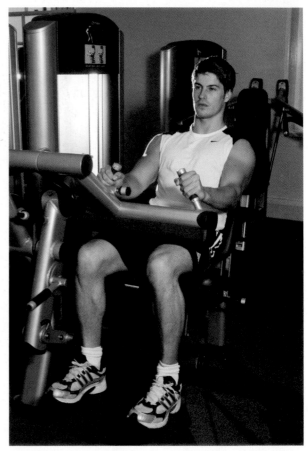

■ Adjust the seat so you are sitting upright or slightly back.
■ Brace your core.
■ Keep looking straight ahead.

■ Pull the pad towards you.
■ Feel the tension in your hamstrings as you return the weights to the start position.

core exercise

---

7 **Swiss ball jackknife**
Targets: abdominals and hip flexors

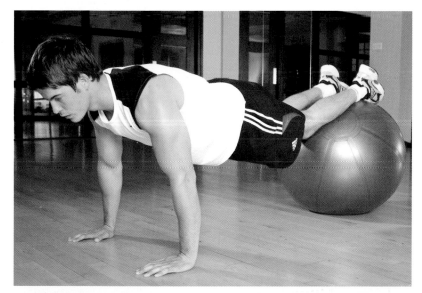

- Place your insteps on ball.
- Keep your body in straight line from head to feet.
- Keep your hands under your shoulders.

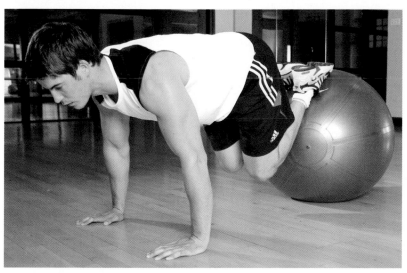

- Pull your feet in towards you.
- Keep your core braced.
- Push your feet away from you and repeat.

Meal plan

Eat these 42 meals to get bigger and stronger

	Monday	**Tuesday**	**Wednesday**	**Thursday**
Breakfast	■ 4 scrambled egg whites on 2 slices of wholemeal toast. ■ Glass of orange juice.	■ Porridge made with 45g oats, 300ml skimmed milk, 1tsp honey and 25g whey protein.	■ 4 scrambled egg whites on 2 slices of wholemeal toast. ■ Glass of orange juice.	■ Porridge made with 45g oats, 300ml skimmed milk, 1tsp honey and 25g whey protein.
Morning snack	■ Mixed nuts, raisins and dried cranberries.	■ 1 mashed banana on 1 slice of wholemeal toast.	■ 120g low-fat yoghurt with blueberries, honey and oats. ■ 1 protein bar.	■ 90g mackerel on 2 slices wholemeal toast. ■ Glass of skimmed milk.
Lunch	■ Turkey and cheese bagel. ■ 1 orange.	■ Turkey salad sandwich on wholemeal bread. ■ 1 orange.	■ Chicken, bacon and avocado baguette. ■ 1 pear.	■ Large jacket potato with tuna, baked beans and grated cheese.
Afternoon snack	■ Smoothie: blend 25g whey protein, 80g raspberries, 80g blueberries and 50g blackberries with 200-300ml water.	■ Mixed nuts, raisins and dried cranberries with cottage cheese.	■ Smoothie: blend 25g whey protein, 100g strawberries and ½ banana with 300ml skimmed milk, and 1tsp flaxseed oil.	■ Smoothie: blend 25g whey protein, 80g raspberries, 80g blueberries and 50g blackberries with 200-300ml water.
Dinner	■ 120g grilled cod with mashed potatoes and peas.	*Italian steak rolls*	■ 120g tuna steak with stir-fried broccoli, cashew nuts, green beans and spinach with sesame oil. ■ 70g brown rice.	■ 90g wholemeal pasta and 200g grilled chicken with jar of tomato sauce and chopped onion.
Bedtime snack	■ Smoothie: blend 25g whey protein, 50g blueberries, 50g blackberries and ½ banana with 300ml skimmed milk.	■ Smoothie: blend 25g whey protein, 50g blueberries, 50g blackberries and ½ banana with 300ml skimmed milk.	■ 100g cottage cheese and pineapple.	■ 120g low-fat yoghurt with strawberries.
Daily totals	■ 2,857 calories ■ 195g protein ■ 345g carbs ■ 66g fat	■ 2,989 calories ■ 210g protein ■ 363g carbs ■ 68g fat	■ 2,922 calories ■ 198g protein ■ 365g carbs ■ 69g fat	■ 2,945 calories ■ 206g protein ■ 367g carbs ■ 69g fat

Friday	Saturday	Sunday
Tropical smoothie ◾ Blend 1 mango, ½ small pineapple, ½ pink grapefruit, 25g whey protein with 200ml water.	◾ Smoothie: blend 25g whey protein, 1 mango, 80g blueberries, 2tbsp natural yoghurt, 1tbsp oats with 100ml apple juice and 100ml water.	◾ 2 scrambled eggs on 2 slices of wholemeal toast. ◾ Glass of orange juice.
◾ 1 mashed banana with 2tbsp peanut butter on 2 slices of wholemeal toast.	◾ 90g sardines with lemon juice on 2 slices of wholemeal toast.	◾ 30g brazil nuts. ◾ Glass of skimmed milk.
◾ Turkey, cheese and mustard bagel. ◾ 1 apple.	◾ Large jacket potato with baked beans and cottage cheese.	◾ Large jacket potato with baked beans, tuna and grated cheese.
◾ 1 tin of tuna with beetroot and cottage cheese.	◾ 140g grilled chicken with beetroot.	◾ Smoothie: blend 25g whey protein, 100g strawberries and ½ banana with 300ml skimmed milk and 1tsp flaxseed oil.
◾ 200g chicken and vegetable stir fry with red and green peppers, cashew nuts, sesame oil and seeds. ◾ 70g brown rice.	◾ 120g fillet steak with mashed potato and spinach.	◾ 150g roast lamb with 100g new potatoes, and mixed vegetables.
◾ Smoothie: blend 25g whey protein, 80g raspberries, 80g blueberries and 50g blackberries with 200-300ml water.	◾ Smoothie: blend 25g whey protein, 80g raspberries, 80g blueberries and 50g blackberries with 200-300ml water.	◾ 100g cottage cheese. ◾ 1 pear.
◾ 2,911 calories ◾ 193g protein ◾ 357g carbs ◾ 68g fat	◾ 2,943 calories ◾ 212g protein ◾ 365g carbs ◾ 69g fat	◾ 3,005 calories ◾ 208g protein ◾ 367g carbs ◾ 74g fat

Italian steak rolls

serves 2

Ingredients
450g fillet steak
2tbs pesto
70g Parma ham
1 large onion, chopped
2 cloves garlic, chopped
1 tin (400g) tomatoes
570ml beef stock

To make
Slice fillet steak and beat slices out thinly. Spread each slice with pesto, sprinkle with ground black pepper, roll up and roll again in a slice of parma ham. If necessary secure each roll with a wooden skewer. Place in a casserole dish and bake in oven at 200°C/400°F/Gas6 for 30 minutes. Remove from oven and place on a plate to rest. Fry onion and garlic in the fat from the casserole until lightly browned. Return the steak rolls, onion and garlic. Mix in the flour and slowly stir in the stock. Add the tomatoes, and seasoning, simmer on a low heat or return to the oven for 1 hour. Serve with green beans dressed with olive oil and ground black pepper, and garlic mash.

Workout log: month 6

See **p101** for sets, reps and times

Theme: High-intensity growth
System: Simple sets
Speed of lift: 1:1
Recovery: 1 minute between sets and exercises

Date: _____

Exercise	Sets	Reps/Time	Weight
Barbell squat			
Barbell split squat			
Seated dumb-bell shoulder press			
Barbell bench press			
Lat pull-down			
Leg curl			
Swiss ball jackknife*			N/A

* Include in 2 of your weekly workouts

Cardio record your sessions below

Workout comments:

Self tests (see p36)

Record your performance below to monitor your progress

Plank endurance

seconds

Lying hamstring stretch

seconds

Press-up

number

Vertical jump

height

Strength

bench kilograms

squat kilograms

(other)

(other)

Measure up

chest

shoulders

thighs

calves

biceps/triceps

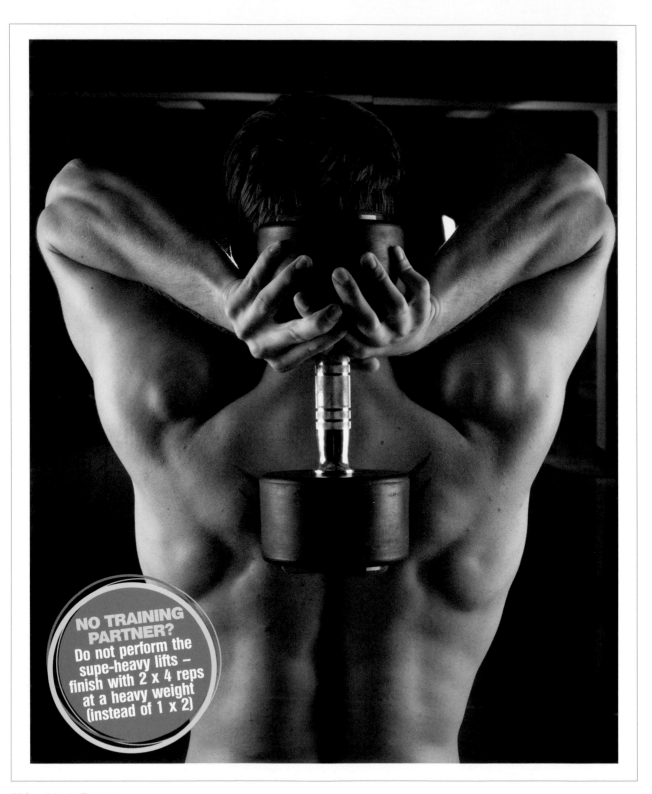

NO TRAINING PARTNER?
Do not perform the supe-heavy lifts – finish with 2 x 4 reps at a heavy weight (instead of 1 x 2)

Ultimate Workout Plan
MONTH 7

AIM to build strength in the eccentric (lowering) phase of lifts

After the intensity of last month, we're going to slow things down a bit – but that doesn't mean you're in for an easy time. We're placing the emphasis on the lowering (eccentric) phase of each lift. So, you'll lift (the concentric contraction) to a one count and lower to a five count. Weights will be near to maximum and, if you have a training partner, above maximum on selected lifts for the last set.

For the four super-heavy eccentric lifts – the bench press, squat, front squat and seated shoulder press – you'll need to use a Smith machine and, on the super heavy set, have a training partner on hand to help you return the weights to the start position. Set the Smith machine up so that if you do get into trouble it will arrest the fall of the weights. This is done by sliding down the catches and positioning them at the bottom-most point of your lift. For the squats this will be when your thighs are parallel to the floor; for the seated shoulder press, this should be when the bar is just below the level of your ears; and for the bench press when the bar is just above your chest.

For the eccentric super-heavy lifts you need to add about ten to 15 per cent of what your actual, or estimated, one-repetition maximum would be on that exercise. After a few workouts you will have gained a feel of what is right.

Month 7:
Eccentric muscle strength

System
Pyramid – with negative reps

Super-heavy eccentric lifts
Bench press
Squat
Seated shoulder press
Front squat

Near super-maximal lifts
Barbell lunge
Lat pull down

Body weight
Pull-up
4 x 6 reps, lower to 5 count.
1 minute between sets.

Core
Side plank with rotation
3 x 10 reps (left and right).
1 minute between sets.

Cardio
1) 1 x 20 minutes easy paced effort
2) 1 complementary interval cardiovascular workout.

Speed of lift
1:5

Rest
2-3 minutes between sets and exercises. More if needed.

Super-heavy eccentric lifts
1 x 8 medium weight
1 x 6 medium/heavy weight
1 x 4 heavy weight
1 x 2 super-heavy weight

Near super-maximal lifts
As above but replace the last set with another 1 x 4 workouts

Week 1
a) Bench press, squat, lunge, pull-up, side plank with rotation
b) Seated shoulder press, front squat, lat pull down
c) Bench press, lunge, pull up

Week 2
a) Front squat, lat pull down, side plank with rotation
b) Squat, bench press, pull-up

Week 3
a) Bench press, squat, lunge, pull-up, side plank with rotation
b) Seated shoulder press, front squat, side plank with rotation, lat pull down
c) Squat, bench press, pull-up

Week 4
a) Bench press, squat, lunge, pull-up, side plank with rotation
b) Seated shoulder press, front squat, lat pull down
c) Bench press, lunge, pull-up

MONTH 7
workout

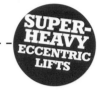

SUPER-HEAVY ECCENTRIC LIFTS

Smith machine eccentric bench press
Targets: pecs

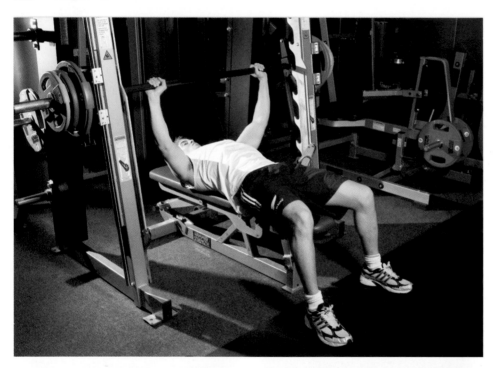

■ Take the bar from the Smith machine.
■ Grip the bar with your hands slightly wider than shoulder-width apart.
■ Hold the bar directly above your chest.
■ Maintain the natural arch of your back.

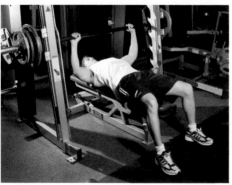

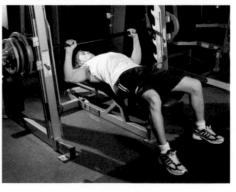

■ Lower to a 5 count.
■ Press back powerfully. You won't be able to do this on the super-heavy lift; your training partner will need to assist you.
■ Don't arch your back.
■ Keep your feet on the floor throughout.

Smith machine eccentric squat

Targets: thighs and glutes

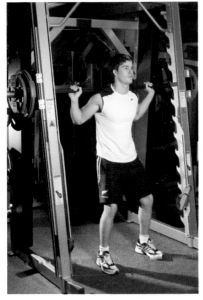

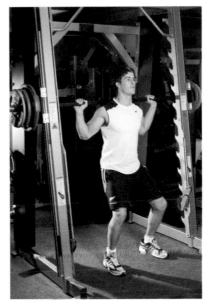

■ Take the bar from the Smith machine and rest it across the fleshy part of your shoulders.
■ Maintain the natural curves of your spine.
■ Feet just beyond hip-width apart.

■ Lower your body until your thighs are parallel to the ground, to a 5 count.
■ Push up through heels. You won't be able to do this on the super-maximal lift. Your training partner will need to assist you. He should support you by squatting behind you and assisting you to lift the bar by lifting you under the arms.
■ Keep looking forward.
■ Maintain the natural curves of your spine.

Smith machine seated eccentric shoulder press

Targets: shoulders

■ Take bar from Smith machine.
■ Brace your core.
■ Keep looking forward.
■ Feet flat on floor.
■ Elbows out.
■ Maintain the your back's natural curves.
■ Lower the bar to a position just above your upper chest.
■ On the super-heavy lift your training partner should assist you to push the bar back up.

MONTH 7
workout

4 Smith machine eccentric front squat

Targets: thighs and backside (emphasis on outer quads)

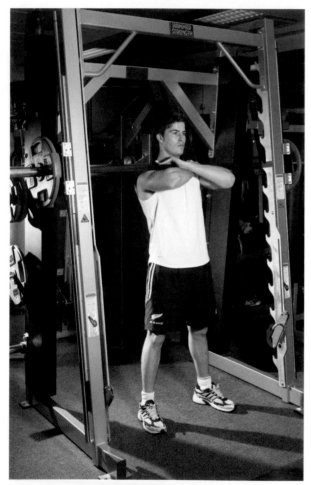

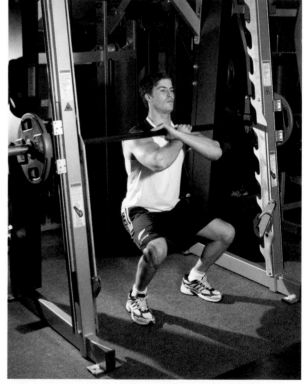

■ Take the bar from the Smith machine and rest it across the fleshy part of the front of shoulders.

■ Keep elbows up and maintain the natural curves of your spine.

■ Feet just beyond hip-width apart.

■ Lower until your thighs are parallel to the ground to a 5 count.

■ Push back up through heels. You won't be able to do this on the super-heavy lift; your training partner will need to assist you. He should support you by squatting behind you and assisting you to lift the bar by lifting you under the arm pits.

■ Keep looking forward.

5 Barbell lunge

Targets: thighs and glutes

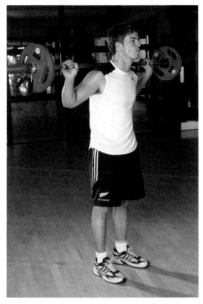

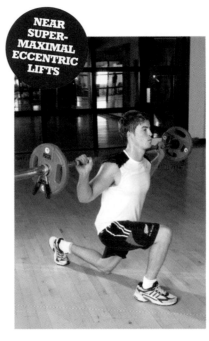

NEAR SUPER-MAXIMAL ECCENTRIC LIFTS

■ Look forward and brace your core.

■ Take a large step forward and place your foot flat on the floor.
■ Keep your torso upright and toes bent under to balance.
■ Don't extend your knee beyond your toes.
■ Lower to a slow 5 count think 'bum to floor' and push back up.
■ Lower your body until your right thigh is parallel to the ground.
■ Complete your designated number of reps and repeat to other side.

6 Lat pull down

Targets: lats and upper back

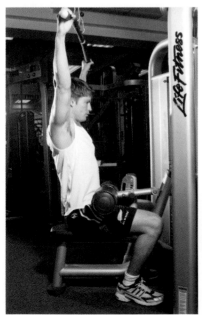

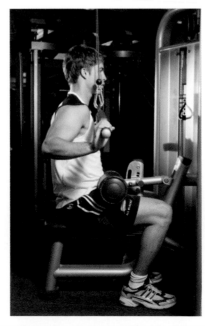

■ Don't lean back too far.
■ Fix your position and back.
■ Look straight ahead.
■ Maintain natural curves of your back.

■ Pull bar down to chest level.
■ Feel your lats release and stretch as you return the bar to the starting position to a 5 count.

MONTH 7
workout

 ### Pull-up
Targets: biceps and lats

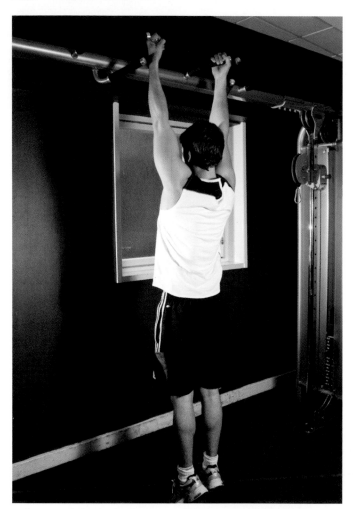

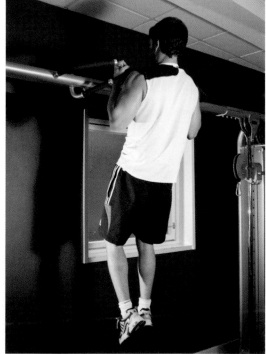

- Use an underhand grip.
- Hands shoulder-width apart.

- Pull up so that your chin is over the bar.
- Don't swing.
- Control the movement.
- Lower to a full extension to a 5 count.

Side plank with rotation
Targets: core

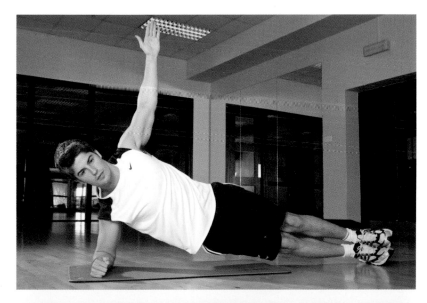

■ Hold your body in a straight line from head to feet.
■ Place your right elbow under your right shoulder.
■ Stack your feet.
■ Lift your left arm up so it is at a right angle to the ground.

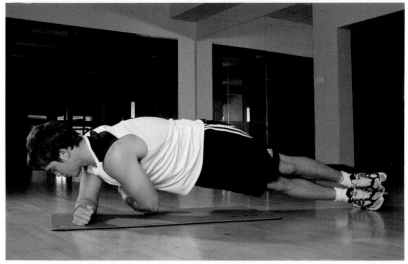

■ Bring your left hand so that it is below your torso rotating your trunk accordingly.
■ Maintain the integrity of the side plank throughout.
■ Complete the designated number of reps and repeat with your right arm.

Meal plan

Pack on lean muscle with this tasty bulk-building menu

	Monday	Tuesday	Wednesday	Thursday
Breakfast	■ 2 scrambled eggs and baked beans on 2 slices of wholemeal toast. ■ Glass of orange juice.	■ Porridge made with 45g oats, 300ml skimmed milk, 1tsp honey and 25g whey protein.	■ 4 scrambled egg whites on 2 slices of wholemeal toast. ■ Glass of orange juice.	■ Porridge made with 45g oats, 300ml skimmed milk, 1tsp honey and 25g whey protein.
morning snack	■ 120g low-fat yoghurt with blueberries, honey and oats. ■ 1 protein bar.	■ 1 mashed banana on 1 slice of of wholemeal toast.	■ Mixed nuts, raisins and dried cranberries.	■ 90g mackerel on 2 slices of wholemeal toast. ■ Glass of skimmed milk.
Lunch	■ Chicken, bacon and avocado baguette. ■ 1 pear.	■ Turkey salad sandwich on wholemeal bread. ■ 1 orange.	■ Turkey and cheese bagel. ■ 1 orange.	■ Smoothie: blend 25g whey protein, 80g raspberries, 80g blueberries and 50g blackberries with 200-300ml water.
Afternoon snack	■ Smoothie: blend 25g whey protein, 100g strawberries and ½ banana with 300ml skimmed milk, and 1tsp flaxseed oil.	■ Mixed nuts, raisins and dried cranberries with cottage cheese.	*Banana and almond smoothie* ■ Blend 25g whey protein, 1 ripe banana, 15g ground almonds and a pinch of ground cinnamon with 300ml skimmed milk.	■ Smoothie: blend 25g whey protein, 100g strawberries and ½ banana with 300ml skimmed milk and 1tsp flaxseed oil.
Dinner	■ 120g tuna steak with stir-fried broccoli, green beans and spinach with sesame oil and seeds. ■ 70g brown rice.	■ Omelette with ham, cheese and tomato.	*Chicken, butternut squash and goat's cheese salad*	■ 150g lean minced-beef chilli with red kidney beans. ■ 70g brown rice.
Bedtime snack	■ 100g cottage cheese and pineapple.	■ Smoothie: blend 25g whey protein, 50g blueberries, 50g blackberries and ½ banana with 300ml skimmed milk.	■ Smoothie: blend 25g whey protein, 50g blueberries, 50g blackberries and ½ banana with 300ml skimmed milk.	■ 120g low-fat yoghurt with strawberries.
Daily totals	■ 2,912 calories ■ 197g protein ■ 365g carbs ■ 67g fat	■ 2,895 calories ■ 201g protein ■ 363g carbs ■ 64g fat	■ 2,857 calories ■ 195g protein ■ 345g carbs ■ 66g fat	■ 2,945 calories ■ 206g protein ■ 367g carbs ■ 69g fat

Friday	Saturday	Sunday
■ Porridge made with 45g oats, 300ml skimmed milk, handful of blueberries, 1tsp honey and 25g whey protein.	■ Smoothie: blend 25g whey protein, 1 mango, 80g blueberries, 2tbsp natural yoghurt, 1tbsp oats with 100ml apple juice and 100ml water.	■ 2 scrambled eggs on 2 slices of wholemeal toast. ■ Glass of orange juice.
■ 1 mashed banana with 2tbsp peanut butter on 2 pieces of wholemeal toast.	■ 90g sardines with lemon juice on 2 slices of wholemeal toast.	■ 30g brazil nuts. ■ Glass of skimmed milk.
■ Turkey, cheese and mustard bagel. ■ 1 apple.	■ Large jacket potato with baked beans and cottage cheese.	■ Large jacket potato with baked beans, tuna and grated cheese.
■ 1 tin of tuna with beetroot and cottage cheese.	■ 140g grilled chicken with beetroot.	■ Smoothie: blend 25g whey protein, 100g strawberries, ½ banana with 300ml skimmed milk and 1tsp flaxseed oil.
■ 120g fillet steak with mashed potato and spinach. ■ Fruit sorbet.	■ 200g chicken and vegetable stir fry with red and green peppers, cashew nuts, sesame oil and seeds. ■ 70g brown rice.	■ 150g roast beef with 100g new potatoes, and mixed vegetables.
■ Smoothie: blend 25g whey protein, 80g raspberries, 80g blueberries and 50g blackberries with 200-300ml water.	■ Smoothie: blend 25g whey protein, 80g raspberries, 80g blueberries and 50g blackberries with 200-300ml water.	■ 100g cottage cheese. ■ 1 apple.
■ 2,950 calories ■ 209g protein ■ 359g carbs ■ 68g fat	■ 2,903 calories ■ 198g protein ■ 365g carbs ■ 69g fat	■ 3,012 calories ■ 211g protein ■ 367g carbs ■ 73g fat

Chicken, butternut squash and goat's cheese salad

serves 2

Ingredients
2 chicken breasts
1 butternut squash
20g goat's cheese
1tbsp olive oil
1tbsp balsamic vinegar
Handful of fresh walnut halves, roughly crushed
Handful of mixed salad leaves
Handful of spinach leaves
Salt and pepper to season

To make
Peel and chop butternut squash into squares, then season and drizzle with olive oil and roast in the oven for 40 minutes. Season and grill the chicken breasts, turning midway, for 20 minutes or until they are fully cooked and the juices run completely clear. Crumble the goat's cheese and walnuts onto the mixed leaves and spinach and serve with the chicken and butternut squash. Add balsamic vinegar for dressing.

Workout log: month 7

See **p113** for sets, reps and times

Theme: Eccentric muscle strength
System: Pyramid with negative reps
Speed of lift: 1:5
Recovery: 2-3 minutes between sets and exercises (more if needed)

Date: _____

Exercise	Sets	Reps/Time	Weight
Smith machine eccentric bench press			
Smith machine eccentric squat			
Smith machine eccentric shoulder press			
Smith machine eccentric front squat			
Barbell lunge			
Lat pull-down			
Pull-up			N/A
Side plank with rotation			N/A

Cardio record your sessions below

Workout comments:

Self tests (see p36)

Record your performance below to monitor your progress

Plank endurance

seconds

Lying hamstring stretch

seconds

Press-up

number

Vertical jump

height

Strength

bench kilograms

squat kilograms

(other)

(other)

Measure up

chest

shoulders

thighs

calves

biceps/triceps

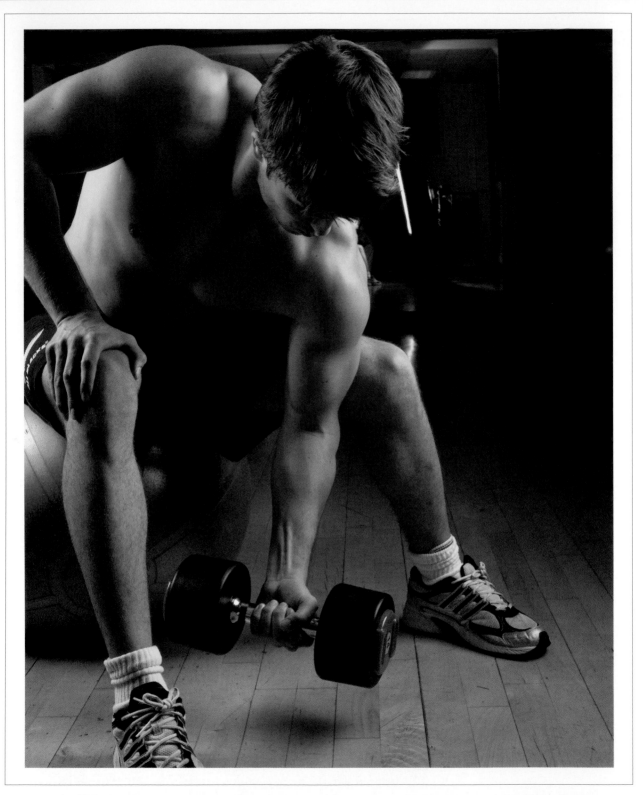

Ultimate Workout Plan
MONTH 8

You'll be pleased to know that this month we're taking a break from the super-heavy weights and are returning to the medium weights. But that doesn't mean you're going to have an easy time. We're not going to lower the intensity, instead you'll be performing multiple sets and reps at a medium weight. This is another growth month. In month six we progressed to 6 x 10 reps, now we go a stage further and move on to 8 x 10.

'You'll be performing multiple reps and sets'

AIM to stimulate muscle growth and hormonal response

Month 8: The growth month

System
Simple sets, medium weights

Bodyweights
Alternate knee-to-shoulder crunch
4 x 30 seconds.
30 seconds recovery.

Pull-up
4 x 12 reps.
1 minute recovery.
2 sessions a week.

Alternate exercises every workout

Free weights
Barbell incline bench press
Barbell front squat
Standing barbell shoulder press
Barbell dead-lift

Fixed weights
Single-leg press
Lat pull down

Cardio
2 complementary cardiovascular
interval training workouts
(see p28)

Workouts

Week 1
a) 5 x 10
b) 5 x 10
c) 4 x 10

Week 2
a) 5 x 12
b) 6 x 10

Week 3
a) 6 x 10
b) 6 x 12
c) 7 x 10

Week 4
a) 7 x 10
b) 8 x 10
c) 8 x 10

Speed of lift
1:2

Rest
2 minutes between sets. Longer
if your form really starts to suffer.

MONTH 8
workout

1 Barbell incline bench press
Targets: upper part of chest (by tilting the bench upward)

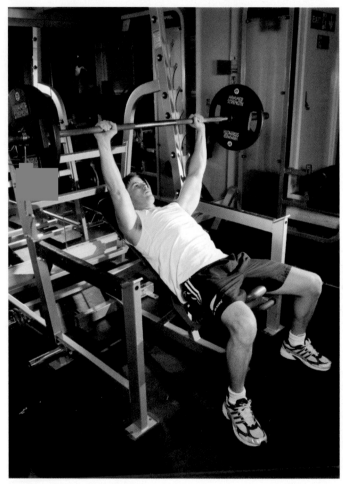

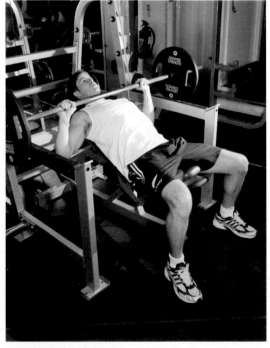

- Incline the bench to 35-40°.
- Take the bar from rack and position it directly above your shoulders.
- Use a grip that's wider than shoulder width.
- Brace your core, but maintain the natural curves of your back.
- Keep feet flat on the floor.

- Lower the bar to chest.
- Don't arch your back.
- Keep your feet on the floor.
- Push back up powerfully.

2 Barbell front squat

Targets: thighs and butt, places more emphasis on the outer quads than back squat

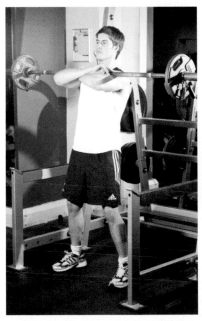

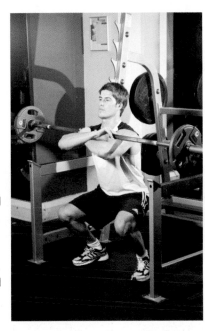

- Take the bar from the rack and rest the it across to top of your upper arms.
- Feet just beyond shoulder-width apart.
- Keep elbows parallel to floor and elbows up.
- Look straight ahead and maintain the natural curves of spine.
- Keep weight pressed through your heels.
- Brace core.

- Lower your torso to a position where your thighs are parallel to the ground.
- Push back up through your heels.
- Keep looking forward throughout the exercise.

3 Standing barbell shoulder press

Targets: deltoids

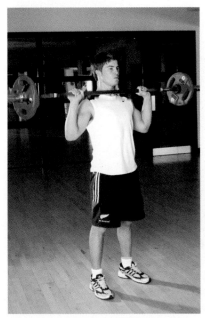

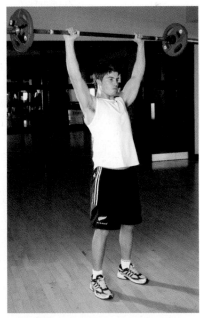

- Look straight ahead.
- Grip the bar with your hands just wider than shoulder width.
- Brace your core.
- Maintain natural curve of spine.
- Keep feet shoulder-width apart.

- Press bar overhead.
- Keep looking forward throughout.
- Keep your core strong and don't arch your back.

MONTH 8
workout

 Barbell deadlift
Targets: back and hamstrings

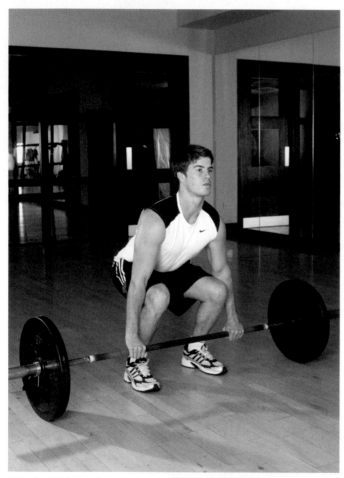

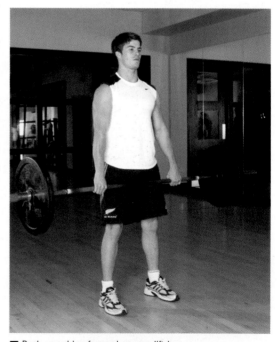

- Look straight head.
- Keep shoulders back.
- Brace your core.
- Maintain the natural curves of your back.

- Feet shoulder-width apart.
- Hold bar with a grip that's slightly wider than shoulder width.
- Sit back and keep the arms long.

- Push your hips forward as you lift bar.
- 'Pull' through your bum and back. Don't squat the bar up.
- Look forward and keep your neck in line with your spine.
- Keep control on bar as you lower.
- Hold your back in position throughout.

Single leg press

Targets: thighs and glutes

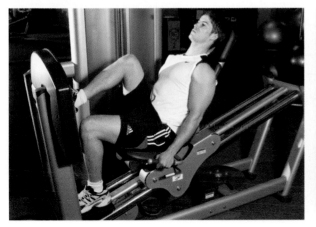

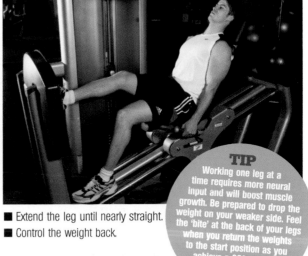

- Look straight ahead.
- Brace your core.
- Place foot to side of centre line of plate.
- Leg aligned through hip, knee and ankle.

- Extend the leg until nearly straight.
- Control the weight back.

TIP
Working one leg at a time requires more neural input and will boost muscle growth. Be prepared to drop the weight on your weaker side. Feel the 'bite' at the back of your legs when you return the weights to the start position as you achieve a 90° angle at your knee joint.

Lat pull down

Targets: lats and upper back

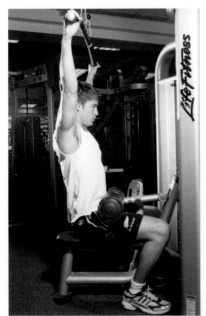

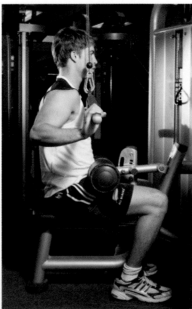

- Don't lean too far back.
- Pull the bar to chest level.
- Fix your position.

- Pull bar down to chest level.
- Feel your lats, release and stretch as you return the bar to the start position,
- Control the movement,

MONTH 8
workout

 Alternate knee-to-shoulder crunch
Targets: abdominals

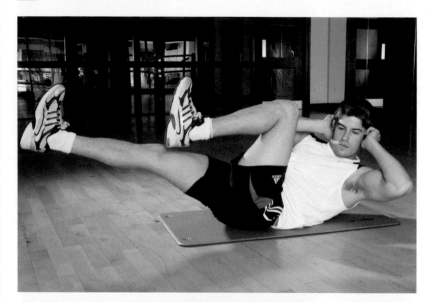

■ Place your hands by your ears.
■ Keep your elbows out.
■ Crunch up and rotate your shoulders.
■ Bring your right elbow to your left knee.

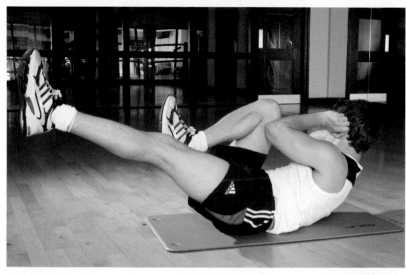

■ Repeat to other side.
■ Control the movement in and out.

8 ▶ Pull-up
Targets: biceps, shoulders and back

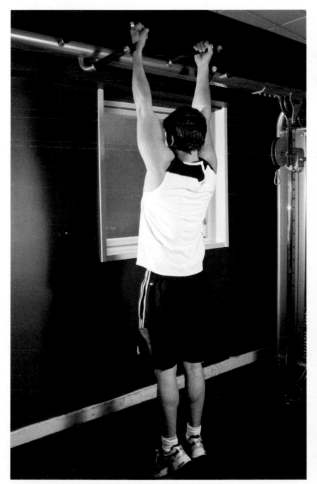

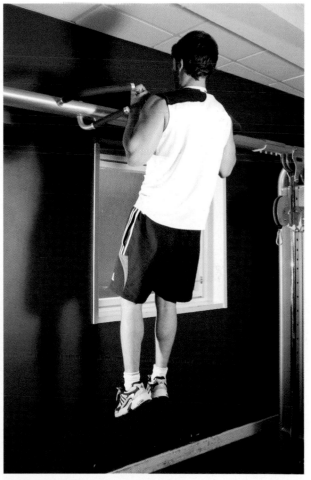

- Underhand grip.
- Hands shoulder-width apart.
- Fully extend your arms.

- Pull up until your chin is over the bar.
- Lower slowly back to start without swinging.

Meal plan

This plan has everything you need to fuel your workouts and get bigger

	Monday	Tuesday	Wednesday	Thursday
Breakfast	■ 4 scrambled egg whites on 2 slices of wholemeal toast. ■ 1 grapefruit.	■ Porridge made with 45g oats, 300ml skimmed milk, 1tsp honey and 25g whey protein.	■ 2 slices French toast made with 1 egg, 1 pint milk, ½tsp cinnamon and ½tsp nutmeg.	■ Porridge made with 45g oats, 300ml skimmed milk, 1tsp honey and 25g whey protein.
Morning snack	■ Mixed nuts, raisins and dried cranberries.	■ 1 mashed banana on 1 slice of wholemeal toast.	■ 120g low-fat yoghurt with blueberries, honey and oats. ■ 1 protein bar.	■ 1 apple with 2tbsp peanut butter. ■ Glass of skimmed milk.
Lunch	■ Turkey and cheese bagel. ■ 1 orange.	■ Turkey salad sandwich on wholemeal bread. ■ 1 apple.	■ Chicken, bacon and avocado baguette. ■ 1 pear.	■ Large jacket potato with tuna, baked beans and grated cheese.
Afternoon snack	■ Smoothie: blend 25g whey protein, 80g strawberries, 80g blueberries and 50g blackberries with 200-300ml water.	■ Mixed nuts, raisins and dried cranberries with cottage cheese.	■ Smoothie: blend 25g whey protein, 100g strawberries and ½ banana with 300ml skimmed milk and 1tsp flaxseed oil.	■ Smoothie: blend 25g whey protein, 80g raspberries, 80g blueberries and 50g blackberries with 200-300ml water.
Dinner	■ 120g salmon with stir-fried broccoli, green beans, red peppers and spinach with sesame oil. ■ 70g brown rice.	**Mandarin and sesame chicken salad**	■ 120g tuna steak with stir-fried broccoli, green beans and spinach with sesame oil and seeds. ■ 70g brown rice.	■ Omelette with ham, cheese, tomato and onion.
Bedtime snack	■ Smoothie: blend 25g whey protein, 50g blueberries, 50g blackberries and ½ banana with 300ml skimmed milk.	■ Smoothie: blend 25g whey protein, 50g blueberries, 50g blackberries and ½ banana with 300ml skimmed milk.	■ 100g cottage cheese and pineapple.	■ 120g low-fat yoghurt with strawberries.
Daily totals	■ 2,857 calories ■ 207g protein ■ 355g carbs ■ 66g fat	■ 2,865 calories ■ 201g protein ■ 363g carbs ■ 64g fat	■ 2,831 calories ■ 211g protein ■ 372g carbs ■ 67g fat	■ 2,887 calories ■ 199g protein ■ 367g carbs ■ 69g fat

Friday	Saturday	Sunday
■ Smoothie: blend 25g whey protein, 1 mango, 80g blueberries, 2tbsp natural yoghurt, 1tbsp oats with 100ml apple juice and 100ml water.	■ Porridge made with 45g oats, 300ml skimmed milk, 1tsp honey and 25g whey protein.	■ 2 scrambled eggs on 2 slices of wholemeal toast. ■ 1 grapefruit. ■ Glass of orange juice.
■ 90g sardines on 2 slices wholemeal toast.	■ 1 mashed banana with 2tbsp peanut butter on 2 slices of wholemeal toast.	■ 30g brazil nuts. ■ Glass of skimmed milk.
■ Medium-sized jacket potato with baked beans and cottage cheese.	■ Turkey, cheese and mustard bagel. ■ 1 apple.	■ Medium-sized jacket potato with baked beans, tuna and grated cheese.
■ 140g grilled chicken with beetroot.	■ 1 tin of tuna with beetroot. ■ 125g low-fat yoghurt.	**Energy smoothie** ■ Blend 25g whey protein, 1 banana and 3 ice cubes with 300ml skimmed milk.
■ 200g chicken and vegetable stir fry with red and green peppers, sesame seeds and oil. ■ 70g brown rice.	■ 120g fillet steak with mashed potato and spinach. ■ Fruit sorbet.	■ 150g roast chicken with 100g new potatoes, and mixed vegetables.
■ Smoothie: blend 25g whey protein, 80g raspberries, 80g blueberries and 50g blackberries with 200-300ml water.	■ Smoothie: blend 25g whey protein, 80g raspberries, 80g blueberries and 50g blackberries with 200-300ml water.	■ 100g cottage cheese. ■ 1 apple.
■ 2,869 calories ■ 212g protein ■ 361g carbs ■ 63g fat	■ 2,950 calories ■ 209g protein ■ 369g carbs ■ 68g fat	■ 2,985 calories ■ 208g protein ■ 362g carbs ■ 73g fat

Mandarin and sesame chicken salad

serves 2

Ingredients
2 chicken breasts
4tbsp sesame oil
2tsp freshly grated ginger
1 garlic clove, crushed
1 red chilli, seeded and finely chopped
Handful of basil and coriander leaves
½ red onion, chopped
150g mange tout
1tsp sesame seeds
5 walnuts, chopped
1 mandarin

To make
Mix 2tbsp sesame oil in a bowl with the garlic, chilli and ginger. Slash the chicken in several places and marinade in the sesame oil mixture for 4 hours. Meanwhile, steam the mange tout for 5 minutes and add to a bowl with the salad leaves, onion, walnuts and sesame seeds. Baste the chicken with the marinade mix and grill for 20 minutes, or until fully cooked and the juices run clear. Cut the chicken into strips and add to the salad. Dress with remainder of the sesame oil and juice of the mandarin.

Workout log: month 8

See **p125** for sets, reps and times

Theme: Growth month

Date: _____

System: Simple sets

Speed of lift: 1:2

Rest: 2 minutes between sets and exercises (longer if form starts to suffer)

Exercise	Sets	Reps/Time	Weight
Barbell incline bench press			
Barbell front squat			
Standing barbell shoulder press			
Barbell deadlift			
Single leg press			
Lat pull-down			
Alternate knee to shoulder crunch			N/A
Pull-up			N/A

Cardio record your sessions below

Workout comments:

Self tests (see p36)

Record your performance below to monitor your progression

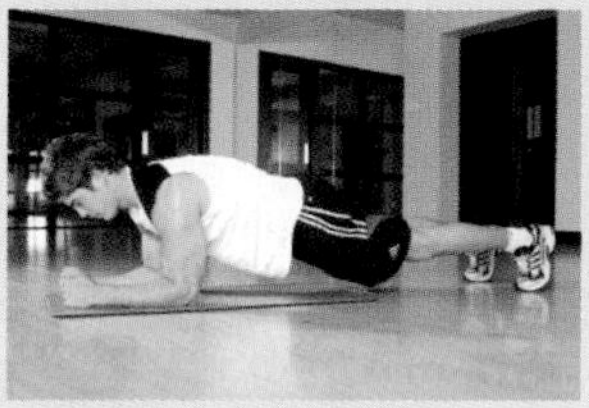

Plank endurance

seconds

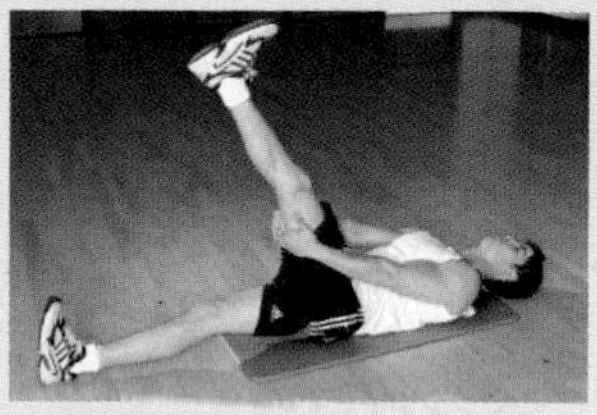

Lying hamstring stretch

seconds

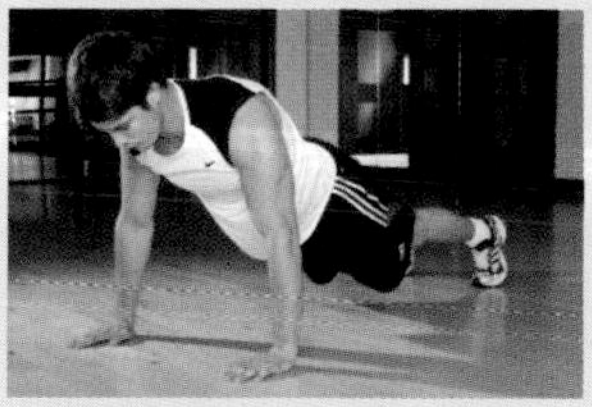

Press-up

number

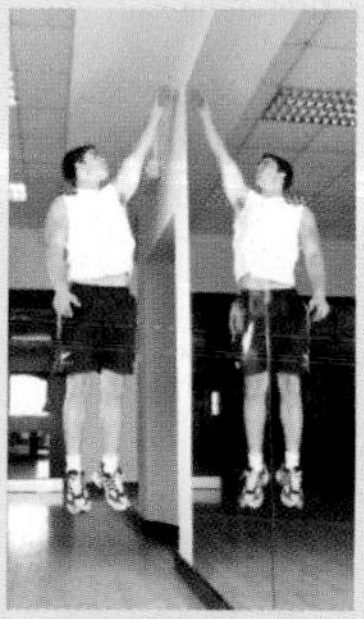

Vertical jump

height

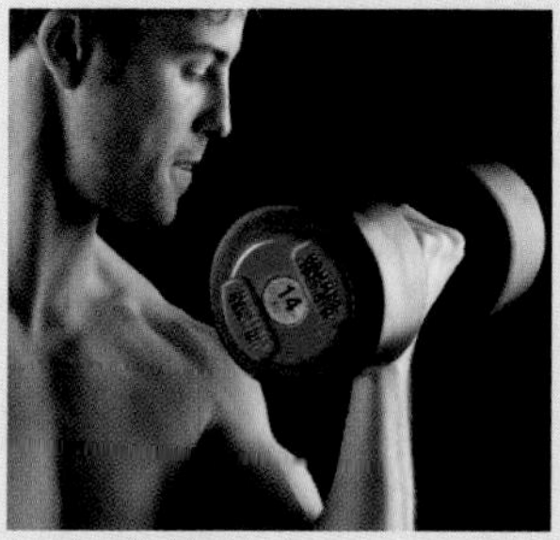

Strength

bench kilograms

squat kilograms

(other)

(other)

Measure up

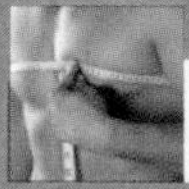

chest

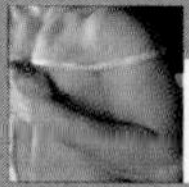

shoulders

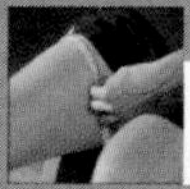

thighs

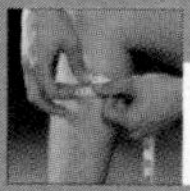

calves

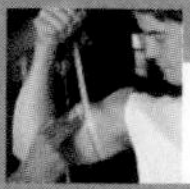

biceps/triceps

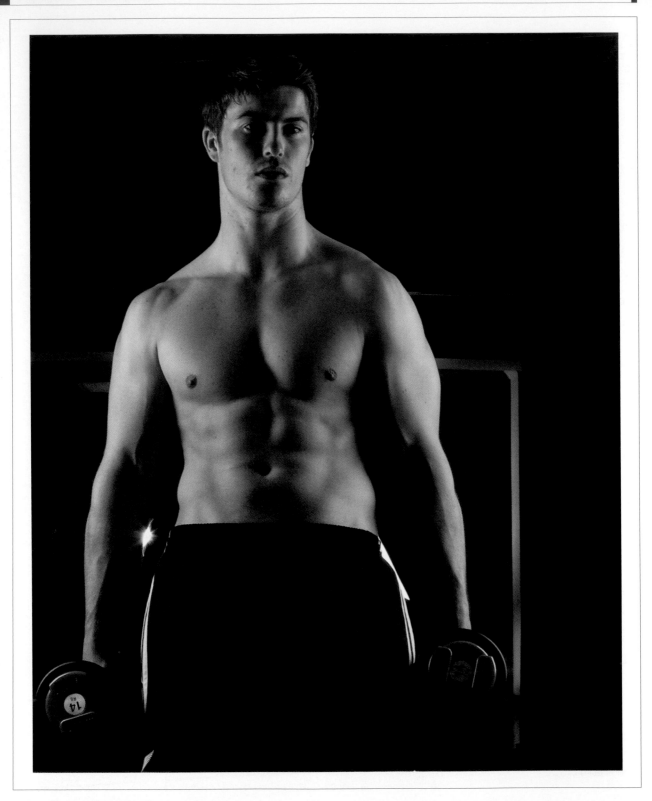

Ultimate Workout Plan

MONTH 9

You've just completed three particularly intense months and now it's time to reduce the intensity slightly to speed up recovery and muscle growth. You'll be lifting light-to-medium weights over multiple simple sets with reasonable recoveries. Repetitions will be high – 20 – and we'll be introducing a more intense workout each week. This will use the superset weight-training system,

'The higher rep supersets will add some definition to your muscles'

which will keep up your high-end strength. Supersets are simply two or more exercises performed back-to-back with no, or minimal, rest in between. This puts your muscles under tension for longer without increasing the length of your workout. Supersets are normally made up of pairs of exercises but in this instance were using supersets of three exercises with relatively low reps. The aim is to build up more endurance in your muscles, which will assist your lower rep, heavier work in the coming months. It's often a lack of endurance, rather than strength that leads to failure at heavier weights and 'last few reps tail-off.

AIM
to develop greater muscular endurance, and provide time for muscle and mind to recover and regenerate

Month 9:
Tone and fat burning

System
Supersets and simple sets

Superset 1 – shoulders
Dumb-bell front raise
Lying reverse lateral raise
Seated dumb-bell shoulder press

Superset 2 – legs
Leg curl
Barbell lunge
Barbell front squat

Superset 3 – chest
Incline dumb-bell flye
Barbell bench press
Press-up

Core exercises
Plank
4 x 45 seconds
(45 seconds recovery)

Seated Russian twist
4 x 20 reps

Alternate exercises each workout.

Simple sets
Select 6 of the above exercises (or other exercises from the *Ultimate Workout Plan*) that work all body parts.

Workouts

Weeks 1-4
2 (endurance) simple sets a week:
4 x 20 light weight

1 (heavy) superset a week.
Alternate supersets each workout, performing 8 reps with a medium/heavy weight on all exercises.

Speed of lift
1:2

Rest:
Supersets
2 minutes between supersets.
Minimum recovery between superset exercises.

Simple sets
1 minute between sets and exercises.

Cardio
1 x easy 20-minute effort.
1 complementary cardiovascular interval training effort (see p28).

MONTH 9
superset 1 - shoulders

1 Dumb-bell front raise

Targets: front of shoulders

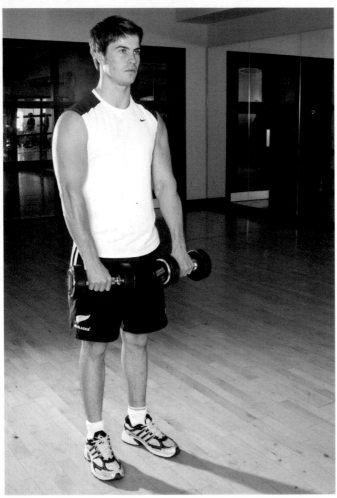

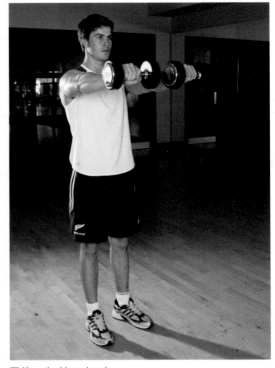

- Stand tall.
- Feet shoulder-width apart.
- Thumbs facing each other.
- Keep your arms long and brace your core.

- Keep looking ahead.
- Lift dumb-bells to shoulder height.
- Lower under control.

2 Lying reverse lateral raise
Targets: rear deltoid

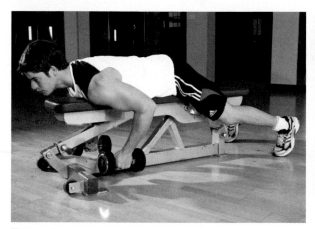
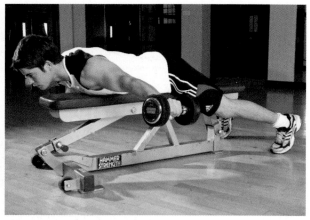

- Keep chest and stomach on bench and look down.
- Keep your toes on the floor for stability.
- Grip dumb-bells below you with palms facing each other.

- Lift weights straight out to the sides.
- Keep arms straight.
- Keep torso in contact with bench.

3 Seated dumb-bell shoulder press
Targets: shoulders

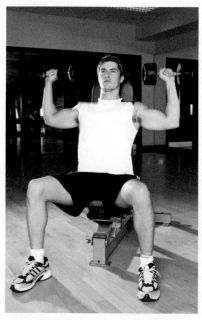

- Look straight ahead and hold the dumb-bells at shoulder-height.
- Keep elbows out to the sides.
- Feet flat on the floor.

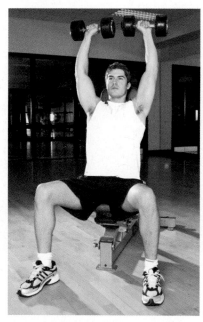

- Don't let the dumb-bells touch at the top of the movement.
- Ensure your core is braced.
- Maintain natural curves of back.

MONTH 9
superset 2 - legs

 Leg curl
Targets: hamstrings

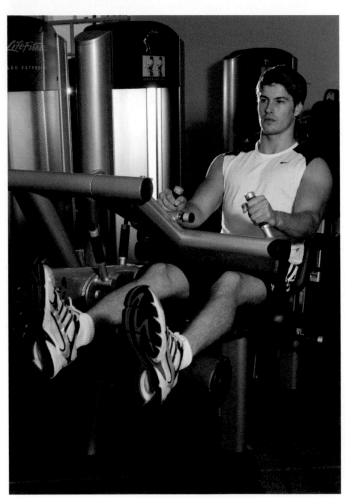

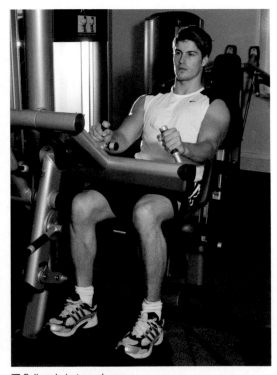

■ Adjust seat so you are sitting upright or slightly back.
■ Brace your core.
■ Look straight ahead.

■ Pull pads in towards you.
■ Focus on controlling the weight back to the start position, feel tension in hamstrings.

Barbell lunge

Targets: thighs and glutes

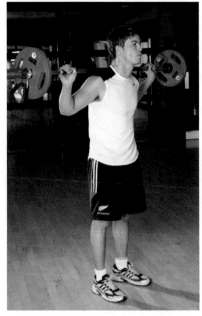

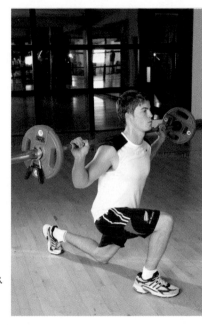

- Rest bar across fleshy part of shoulders.
- Look forward and brace your core.

- Take a large step forward.
- Place foot flat on the floor.
- Keep torso upright.
- Toes bent under to balance.
- Don't extend knee forward of ankle.
- Lower until your thigh is parallel to the floor and push back up.

Barbell front squat

Targets: thighs and glutes (throws more emphasis onto quads, particularly the outer portion, than back squat)

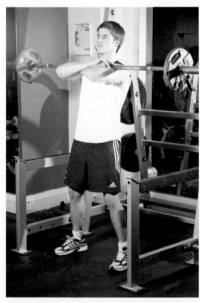

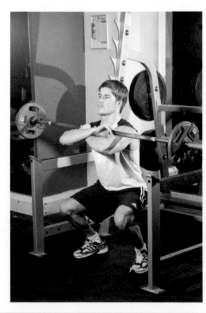

- Take the bar from the rack and rest it across your shoulders.
- Keep upper arms parallel to the floor.
- Maintain the natural curves of your spine.
- Feet just beyond hip-width apart and keep looking forward.

- Lower until your thighs are parallel to the ground.
- Push back up through your heels.
- Keep looking forward.
- Maintain the natural curves of your spine.

MONTH 9
superset 3 - chest

1 Incline dumb-bell flye
Targets: places emphasis on upper pecs

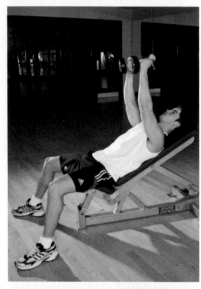

■ Angle the bench to 30-45°.
■ Hold the dumb-bells directly above your chest.
■ Keep your feet flat on floor.

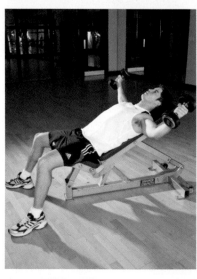

■ Lower the dumb-bells in an arc out to the sides.
■ Focus on pecs to pull weights back to start position.
■ Maintain slight bend in elbows.

2 Barbell bench press
Targets: pecs, deltoids and triceps

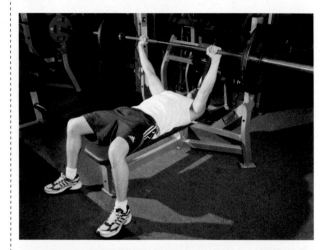

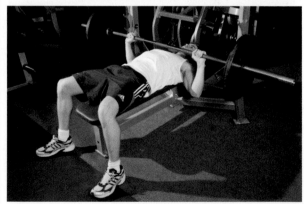

■ Brace your core and keep your head and shoulders on the bench.
■ Maintain the natural curves of your back.
■ Keep your feet on the floor.
■ Lower weights under control.
■ Push weight back powerfully.
■ Push evenly through both arms.
■ Do not arch your back as you press.

3 Press-up
Targets: chest, shoulders and triceps

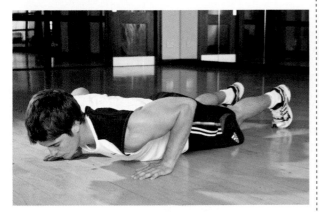

- Keep body in a straight line from head to toe.
- Brace your core.
- Point elbows back.
- Lower your body, not your chest.

1 Plank
Targets: core

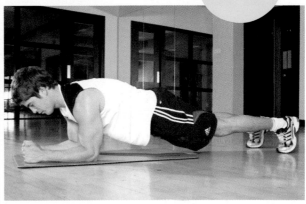

core exercise

- Look down.
- Maintain head in alignment with your body.
- Place your elbows beneath your shoulders.
- Relax in the held position.

2 Seated Russian twist
Targets: abdominals

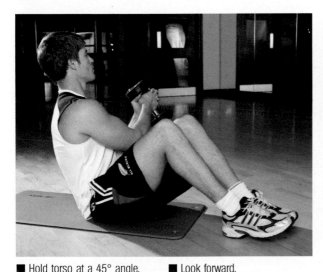

- Hold torso at a 45° angle.
- Hold dumb-bell in both hands at chest height.
- Keep knees bent at 90°.
- Look forward.
- Twist to one side.

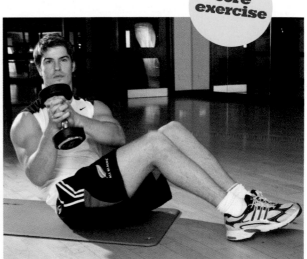

core exercise

- Maintain body angle.
- Twist to other side.
- Focus on your abs and control the movement with them.

Meal plan

With around 3,000 calories a day, this plan will help you add lean muscle

	Monday	Tuesday	Wednesday	Thursday
Breakfast	■ 4 scrambled egg whites on 2 slices of wholemeal toast. ■ 1 grapefruit.	■ Porridge made with 45g oats, 300ml skimmed milk, 1tsp honey and 25g whey protein.	■ 2 slices of French toast made with 1 egg, 1 pint milk, ½tsp cinnamon and ½tsp nutmeg.	■ 2 scrambled eggs on 2 slices of wholemeal toast. ■ Glass of orange juice.
Morning snack	■ Mixed nuts, raisins and dried cranberries.	■ 1 apple with 2tbsp peanut butter. ■ Glass of skimmed milk.	■ 120g low-fat yoghurt with blueberries, honey and oats. ■ 1 protein bar.	■ 1 mashed banana on 1 slice of wholemeal toast. ■ 1 protein bar.
Lunch	■ Turkey and cheese salad sandwich on wholemeal bread. ■ 1 pear.	■ Medium-sized jacket potato with tuna, baked beans and grated cheese.	■ Turkey and cranberry wholemeal sandwich. ■ 1 pear.	■ Turkey salad sandwich on wholemeal bread. ■ 1 apple.
Afternoon snack	*Berry blast smoothie* ■ Blend 25g whey protein, 50g strawberries, 50g raspberries, 50g blueberries and 50g blackberries with water.	■ Smoothie: blend 25g whey protein, 80g raspberries, 80g blueberries and 50g blackberries with 200-300ml water.	■ Smoothie: blend 25g whey protein, 100g strawberries and ½ banana with 300ml skimmed milk and 1tsp flaxseed oil.	■ Mixed nuts, raisins and dried cranberries with cottage cheese.
Dinner	■ 200g chicken and vegetable stir fry with red and green peppers, sesame seeds and oil. ■ 70g brown rice.	■ 120g fillet steak with mashed potato and spinach. ■ Slice of cheesecake.	■ 150g lean minced-beef chilli with kidney beans. ■ 70g brown rice.	*Moroccan chicken*
Bedtime snack	■ Smoothie: blend 25g whey protein, 50g blueberries, 50g blackberries and ½ banana with 300ml skimmed milk.	■ 120g low-fat yoghurt with strawberries.	■ 100g cottage cheese and pineapple.	■ Smoothie: blend 25g whey protein, 50g blueberries, 50g blackberries and ½ banana with 300ml skimmed milk.
Daily totals	■ 2,847 calories ■ 211g protein ■ 345g carbs ■ 65g fat	■ 2,976 calories ■ 212g protein ■ 355g carbs ■ 73g fat	■ 2,834 calories ■ 207g protein ■ 362g carbs ■ 67g fat	■ 2,835 calories ■ 211g protein ■ 352g carbs ■ 62g fat

serves 2

Friday	Saturday	Sunday
■ Smoothie: blend 25g whey protein, 1 mango, 80g blueberries, 2tbsp yoghurt, 1tbsp oats with100ml apple juice and 100ml water.	■ Porridge made with 45g oats, 300ml skimmed milk, 1tsp honey and 25g whey protein.	■ 2 scrambled eggs and 2 rashers of bacon on 2 slices of wholemeal toast. ■ 1 grapefruit. ■ Glass of orange juice.
■ 90g sardines on 2 slices wholemeal toast.	■ 1 mashed banana with 2tbsp peanut butter on 2 slices of wholemeal toast.	■ 30g brazil nuts. ■ Glass of skimmed milk.
■ Medium-sized jacket potato with baked beans and cottage cheese.	■ Turkey, cheese and mustard bagel. ■ 1 apple.	■ Medium-sized jacket potato with baked beans and cottage cheese.
■ 140g grilled chicken with beetroot.	■ 1 tin of tuna with beetroot. ■ 125g low-fat yoghurt.	■ Smoothie: blend 25g whey protein, 80g raspberries, 80g blueberries and 50g blackberries with water.
■ 120g tuna steak with stir-fried broccoli, green beans and spinach with sesame oil and seeds. ■ 70g brown rice.	■ 120g grilled cod, mashed potato and peas.	■ 150g roast pork with 100g new potatoes, and mixed vegetables.
■ Smoothie: blend 25g whey protein, 80g raspberries, 80g blueberries and 50g blackberries with 200-300ml water.	■ Smoothie: blend 25g whey protein, 80g raspberries, 80g blueberries and 50g blackberries with 200-300ml water.	■ Smoothie: blend 25g whey protein, 100g strawberries and ½ banana with 300ml skimmed milk and 1tsp flaxseed oil.
■ **2,910 calories** ■ **212g protein** ■ **351g carbs** ■ **63g fat**	■ **2,923 calories** ■ **205g protein** ■ **359g carbs** ■ **68g fat**	■ **3,016 calories** ■ **212g protein** ■ **364g carbs** ■ **73g fat**

Moroccan chicken

Ingredients
4 chicken breasts
2 garlic cloves, crushed
1 red chilli, seeded
and sliced
½ lemon
100g couscous
100g tinned chick peas
100g tinned apricots
Pinch of paprika
Pinch of cumin

To make
Mix together the juice and zest of the lemon, garlic, chilli, paprika and cumin, and place to one side in a bowl. Slash the chicken breasts in three places and marinade in the lemon mixture for 4 hours. Soak the couscous in boiling water for 15 minutes, then add the chick peas and apricots. Meanwhile grill the chicken breasts for 20 minutes or until they are fully cooked and the juices run clear, turning halfway through. Serve with the couscous.

Workout log: month 9

See for sets, reps and times

Theme: Tone and fat burning
Date: _____

System: Simple sets and supersets
Speed of lift: 1:2
Rest: 2 minutes between supersets, 2 minutes recovery between simple-set exercises

Exercise	Sets	Reps/Time	Weight
Superset 1 – shoulders			
Dumb-bell front raise			
Lying reverse dumb-bell lateral raise			
Seated dumb-bell shoulder press			
Superset 2 – legs			
Leg curl			
Barbell lunge			
Barbell front squat			
Superset 3 – chest			
Incline dumb-bell flye			
Barbell bench press			
Press-up			
Core			
Plank			N/A
Seated Russian twist			

Cardio record your sessions below

Workout comments:

Self tests (see p36)

Record your performance below to monitor your progress

Plank endurance

seconds

Lying hamstring stretch

seconds

Press-up

number

Vertical jump

height

Strength

bench kilograms

squat kilograms

(other)

(other)

Measure up

chest

shoulders

thighs

calves

biceps/triceps

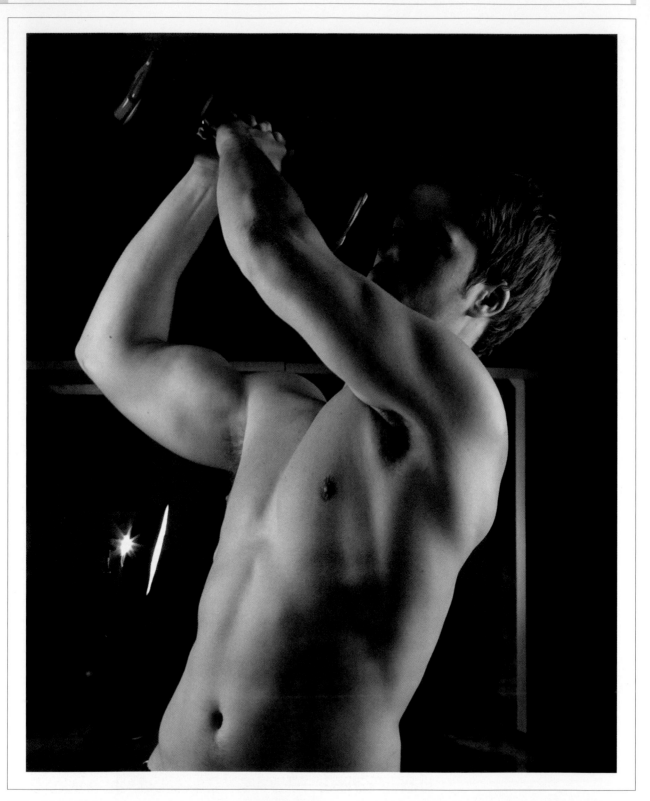

Ultimate Workout Plan
MONTH 10

AIM to stimulate further growth by using the very intense drop-set system

To keep your mind and your muscles on their toes we're going to introduce another new system of training in the *Ultimate Workout Plan* this month: drop sets. We've included four variants in this monthly plan, simply alternate these session by session, week by week. Drop sets are tough. You max out on every set in terms of repetitions, the only concession being that you use a lighter

'One of the simplest ways to do drop sets is with dumb-bells'

weight for each set (where applicable). Don't worry exactly about the weight to use – you'll get a feel and all you have to do is rep out!

One of the simplest ways to perform drop sets is to use dumb-bells. This way you simply 'run the rack' using a lighter pair for each set.

We've also included some bodyweight exercises, such as the wide-grip pull-up, and for these you simply need to complete as many reps as you can for each set.

Month 10: Growth month

System
Drop sets

Drop set 1
Dumb-bell bench press
Dumb-bell squat
Standing dumb-bell shoulder press

Drop set 2
Incline bench press
Dumb-bell lunge
Dumb-bell lateral lift

Drop set 3
Wide-grip pull-up
Dumb-bell bicep curl
Barbell step-up

Drop set 4
Lat pull-down
Barbell split squat
Cable crossover flye

Cardio
2 x easy paced 20-minute efforts

Workouts

Weeks 1-4
Perform a different drop-set workout each workout. Start with a medium/heavy weight and use lighter dumb-bells/weights for each of the subsequent 5 sets, until you're lifting a very light weight.
Perform 3 workouts a week.

Speed of lift
1:2

Rest
3 minutes between drop-set exercises.

Bodyweight exercises
Perform 5 sets with 10 seconds recovery, going for maximum number of reps each time.

MONTH 10
drop set 1

 Dumb-bell bench press
Targets: pectorals, deltoids and triceps

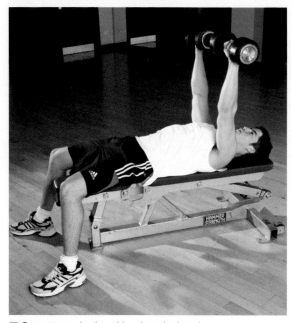

- Support your back and head on the bench.
- Maintain the natural curves of your back.
- Hold dumb-bells with thumbs facing each other,
- Hold dumb-bells at chest level.
- Press the dumb-bells up over your shoulders.
- Keep your feet on the floor.
- Don't arch your back.
- Control the movement down.

2 **Dumb-bell squat**
Targets: thighs and glutes

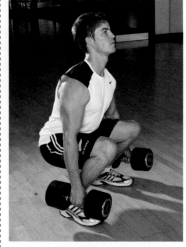

- Look straight ahead.
- Hold the dumb-bells at arms' length.
- Feet flat on the floor.
- Ensure core is braced.
- Maintain natural curves of your back.
- Lower until your thighs are parallel to the ground.
- Push back up through your heels.

3 **Standing dumb-bell shoulder press**
Targets: shoulders

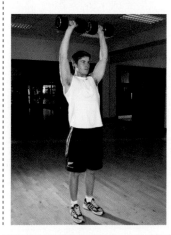

- Look straight ahead.
- Hold the dumb-bells at shoulder-height.
- Keep elbows out to the sides.
- Push the dumb-bells above your head.
- Don't let the dumb-bells touch at the top of the movement.
- Ensure core is braced.
- Maintain natural curves of your back.

drop set 2

1 Incline bench press

Targets: upper part of chest by tilting the bench upward

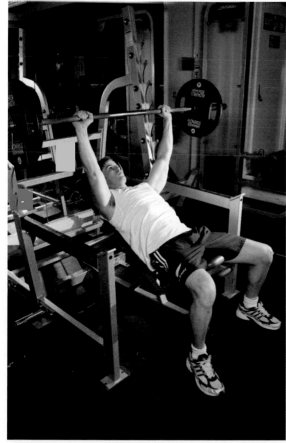

- Incline the bench to a 35-40° angle.
- Keep your feet flat on the floor.
- Grip the bar with hands wider than shoulder-width apart.
- Take the bar from rack and position directly over shoulders.
- Brace your core, but maintain the natural curves of your back.
- Lower the bar to chest.
- Push back up.

2 Dumb-bell lunge

Targets: thighs and glutes

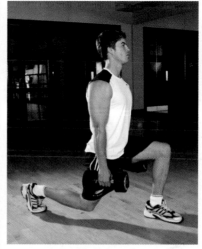

- Take a large step forward, place foot flat on the ground.
- Don't extend your knee past your toes.
- Keep your chest up.
- Bend front knee until thigh is at right angles to the ground.
- Lower back knee until it almost contacts the ground.
- Push back powerfully.

3 Dumb-bell lateral lift

Targets: side deltoids

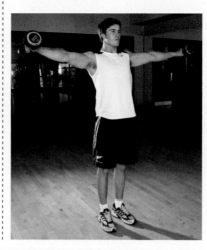

- Look straight ahead.
- Maintain the natural curves of your spine.
- Feet just beyond shoulder-width apart.
- Hold dumb-bells at arms' length.
- Lift to shoulder height.
- Keep your core braced.
- Control weights down.

MONTH 10
drop set 3

1 Wide-grip pull-up

Targets: shoulders and back (places more emphasis on lats)

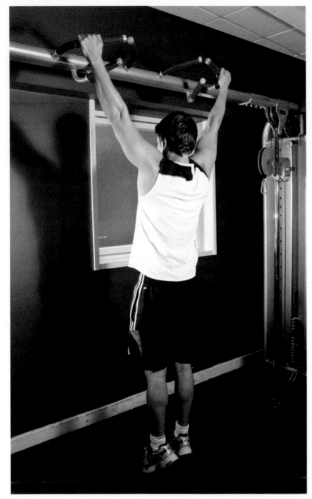

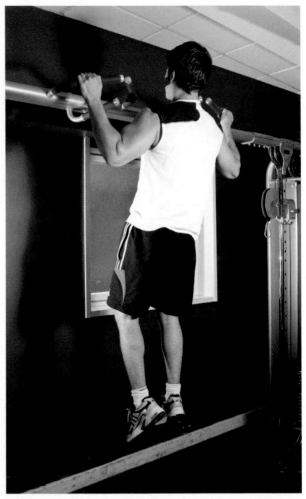

- Use an over-hand grip.
- Grip the bar with your hands beyond shoulder-width apart
- Extend your arms fully in the down position.
- Keep your body still.

- Squeeze your lats as you pull up.
- Pull up until your chin is over the bar.
- Lower under control without swinging.

Dumb-bell biceps curl
Targets: biceps

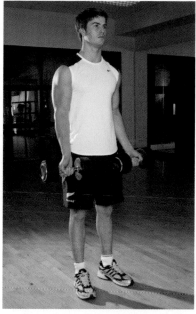

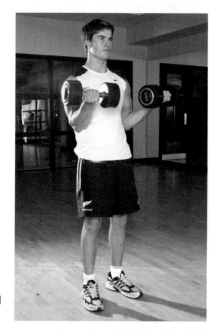

■ Stand with feet shoulder-width apart and thumbs facing each other.
■ Look straight ahead and brace your core.

■ Curl the dumb-bells to chest height while keeping your elbows 'pinned' to your sides.
■ Lower dumb-bells under control.
■ Do not swing dumb-bells when the going gets tough.

Barbell step-up
Targets: legs and backside

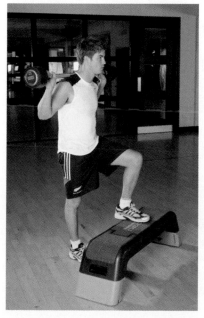

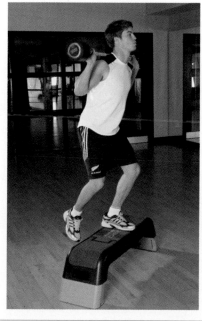

■ Look straight ahead.
■ Rest bar across the fleshy part of your shoulders.
■ Place your foot firmly on the step.

■ Push up through foot.
■ Push hips forward.
■ Keep back braced
■ Bring back leg up to join lead leg.
■ Step back down with same leg.
■ Alternate legs.

MONTH 10
drop set 4

- -

Lat pull-down
Targets: lats, upper back

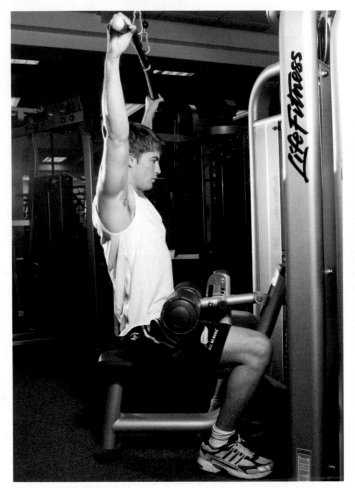

- Don't lean back too far.
- Brace your core.

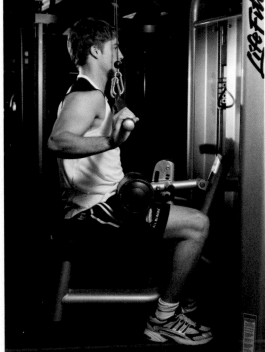

- Pull the bar to mid chest level.
- Fix your position and 'feel' your lats work.
- Feel your lats release and stretch as you return the bar to the start position.
- Control the movement.

2 Barbell split squat
Targets: thighs and glutes

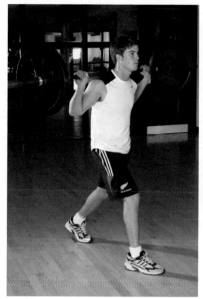

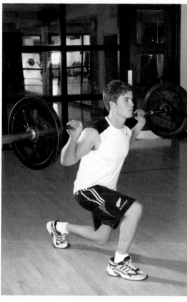

- Support the bar on the fleshy part of your shoulders.
- Look straight ahead and take a large step forward with your right foot.
- Brace your core and keep your knee behind your toes.
- Support the weight on the toes of your left foot.
- Maintain the natural curves of your back.

- Bend your left knee to lower your body until your right thigh is parallel to the ground.
- Think 'bum to floor'.
- Straighten your left leg to return to the start position.
- Complete your designated number of repetitions with your right leg forward and then repeat with your left leg forward.

3 Cable crossover flye
Targets: pecs

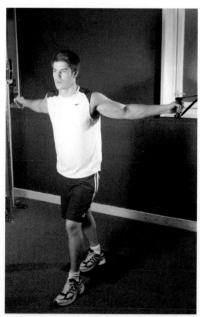

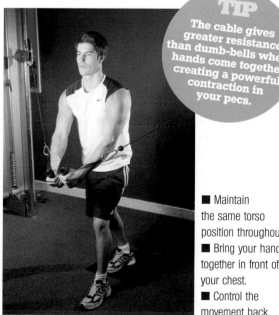

TIP
The cable gives greater resistance than dumb-bells where hands come together creating a powerful contraction in your pecs.

- Use a split stance for stability.
- Position the pulleys so that you grip the cable attachment at approximately shoulder height.
- Brace your core.
- Look straight ahead.

- Maintain the same torso position throughout.
- Bring your hands together in front of your chest.
- Control the movement back.

Meal plan

Use this high-protein meal plan to complement your training

	Monday	Tuesday	Wednesday	Thursday
Breakfast	■ Porridge made with 45g oats, 300ml skimmed milk, 1tsp honey and 25g whey protein.	■ 2 scrambled eggs and baked beans on 2 slices of wholemeal toast. ■ Glass of orange juice.	■ 4 scrambled egg whites on 2 slices of wholemeal toast. ■ Glass of orange juice.	■ Porridge made with 45g oats, 300ml skimmed milk, 1tsp honey and 25g whey protein.
Morning snack	■ 1 mashed banana on 1 slice of wholemeal toast.	■ 120g low-fat yoghurt with blueberries, honey and oats. ■ 1 protein bar.	■ Mixed nuts, raisins and dried cranberries.	■ 90g mackerel on 2 slices wholemeal toast. ■ Glass of skimmed milk.
Lunch	■ Turkey salad sandwich on wholemeal bread. ■ 1 orange.	■ Chicken, bacon and avocado baguette. ■ 1 pear.	■ Turkey and cheese bagel. ■ 1 orange.	■ Large jacket potato with tuna, baked beans and grated cheese.
Afternoon snack	■ Mixed nuts, raisins and dried cranberries with cottage cheese.	■ Smoothie: blend 25g whey protein, 100g strawberries and ½ banana with 300ml skimmed milk and 1tsp flaxseed oil.	**Banana, apple and cinnamon smoothie** ■ Blend 25g whey protein, 50g natural yoghurt, 1 ripe banana, 1 apple and a pinch of ground cinnamon with 200ml skimmed milk.	■ Smoothie: blend 25g whey protein, 80g raspberries, 80g blueberries and 50g blackberries blend with water.
Dinner	**Chicken stir-fry**	■ 120g tuna steak with stir-fried broccoli, green beans and spinach with sesame oil and seeds. ■ 70g brown rice.	■ 120g salmon with stir-fried broccoli, green beans, red peppers and spinach with sesame oil. ■ 70g brown rice.	■ 150g lean minced-beef chilli with kidney beans. ■ 70g brown rice.
Bedtime snack	■ Smoothie: blend 25g whey protein, 50g blueberries, 50g blackberries and ½ banana with 300ml skimmed milk.	■ 100g cottage cheese and pineapple.	■ Smoothie: blend 25g whey protein, 50g blueberries, 50g blackberries and ½ banana with 300ml skimmed milk.	■ 120g low-fat yoghurt with strawberries.
Daily totals	■ 2,895 calories ■ 201g protein ■ 363g carbs ■ 64g fat	■ 2,912 calories ■ 197g protein ■ 365g carbs ■ 67g fat	■ 2,875 calories ■ 195g protein ■ 345g carbs ■ 66g fat	■ 2,945 calories ■ 206g protein ■ 367g carbs ■ 69g fat

Friday	Saturday	Sunday
■ Porridge made with 45g oats, 300ml skimmed milk, handful of blueberries 1tsp honey, and 25g whey protein.	■ Smoothie: blend 25g whey protein, 1 mango, 80g blueberries, 2tbsp natural yoghurt and 1tbsp oats with 100ml apple juice and 100ml water.	■ 2 scrambled eggs on 2 slices of wholemeal toast. ■ Glass of orange juice.
■ 1 mashed banana with 2tbsp peanut butter on 2 slices of wholemeal toast.	■ 90g sardines with lemon juice on 2 slices of wholemeal toast.	■ 30g brazil nuts. ■ Glass of skimmed milk.
■ Turkey, cheese and mustard bagel. ■ 1 apple.	■ Large jacket potato with baked beans and cottage cheese.	■ Large jacket potato with baked beans, tuna and grated cheese.
■ 1 tin of tuna with beetroot and cottage cheese.	■ 140g grilled chicken with beetroot.	■ Smoothie: blend 25g whey protein, 100g strawberries and ½ banana with 300ml skimmed milk and 1tsp flaxseed oil.
■ 120g fillet steak with mashed potato and spinach. ■ Fruit sorbet.	■ 200g chicken and vegetable stir fry with red and green peppers, cashew nuts, sesame oil and seeds. ■ 70g brown rice.	■ 150g roast beef with 100g new potatoes, and mixed vegetables.
■ Smoothie: blend 25g whey protein, 80g raspberries, 80g blueberries and 50g blackberries with 200-300ml water.	■ Smoothie: blend 25g whey protein, 80g raspberries, 80g blueberries and 50g blackberries with 200-300ml water.	■ 100g cottage cheese. ■ 1 apple.
■ 2,950 calories ■ 210g protein ■ 359g carbs ■ 68g fat	■ 2,903 calories ■ 198g protein ■ 365g carbs ■ 69g fat	■ 3,012 calories ■ 209g protein ■ 367g carbs ■ 73g fat

serves 2

Chicken stir-fry

Ingredients
2 chicken breasts
5 cauliflower florets
3 tomatoes, chopped
5 olives, chopped
½ red pepper, sliced
½ green pepper, sliced
½tsp fresh rosemary, finely chopped
1tsp fresh thyme, finely chopped
1tbsp sesame oil
1tsp sesame seeds
Pinch of black pepper

To make
Steam the cauliflower florets for 5 minutes and place to one side. Heat a wok or a large non-stick frying pan over a medium heat and coat the bottom with the sesame oil. Cut chicken into strips and place in pan for 6-7 minutes, until fully cooked. Add the steamed cauliflower, tomatoes, peppers, herbs and pepper, and cook for an additional 3 minutes. Add the olives and sesame seeds and then cook for a further 1 minute. Serve with 70g of brown rice.

Workout log: month 10

See **p149** for sets, reps and times

Theme: Growth month
System: Drop sets
Speed of lift: 1:2
Rest: 3 minutes between drop sets

Date: _____

Exercise	Sets	Reps/Time	Weight
Perform one of the 4 different drop sets each workout			
Drop set 1			
Dumb-bell bench press			
Dumb-bell squat			
Standing dumb-bell shoulder press			
Drop set 2			
Incline bench press			
Dumb-bell lunge			
Dumb-bell lateral lift			
Drop set 3			
Wide-grip pull-up			
Dumb-bell biceps curl			
Barbell step-up			
Drop set 4			
Lat pull-down			
Barbell split squat			
Cable crossover flye			

Cardio record your sessions below

Workout comments:

Self tests (see p36)

Record your performance below to monitor your progress

Plank endurance

seconds

Lying hamstring stretch

seconds

Press-up

number

Vertical jump

height

Strength

bench kilograms

squat kilograms

(other)

(other)

Measure up

chest

shoulders

thighs

calves

biceps/triceps

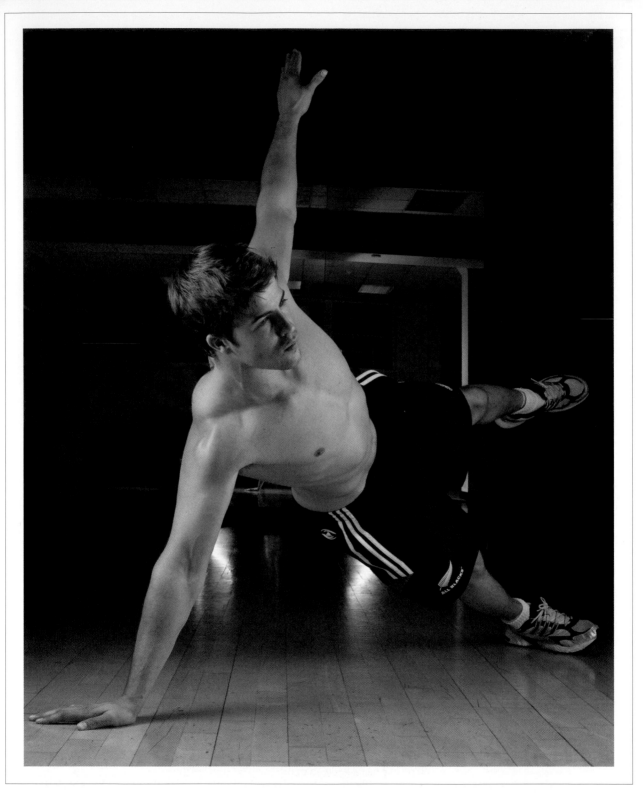

Ultimate Workout Plan
MONTH 11

As the *Ultimate Workout Plan* nears its end we continue to build muscle with some more muscle shock tactics, using the pre-exhaust system. Pre-exhaust weight training is extremely demanding, but very effective in promoting greater gains in muscle size, power and strength. The idea is that you exhaust a muscle with an isolation move first, then you continue to work the fatigued muscle in the compound exercise. This adds up to more muscle fibre recruitment, more hormonal

'Pre-exhaust weight training is very demanding'

stimulation and to greater size, power and strength gains.

This month we've also included unilateral lifts, such as the one-arm dumb-bell overhead press. This will have the effect of further stimulating muscle growth, preventing boredom and promoting more symmetrical strength and muscle development.

Month 11:

System
Pre-exhaust

Pre-exhaust set 1
Bench triceps dip
Barbell bench press

Pre-exhaust set 2
Leg extension
Barbell squat

Pre-exhaust set 3
Dumb-bell lateral raise
One-arm dumb-bell overhead press

Pre-exhaust set 4
Leg curl
Leg press

Pre-exhaust set 5
One-leg squat
Front squat

Core
Plank
4 x 1 minute holds
15-second recovery between holds.
Crunch
4 x 15 reps
1 minute recovery between sets
Perform twice a week.

Cardio
2 x complementary cardiovascular interval sessions (see p28).

Workouts
12 reps medium weight first exercise (where applicable)
5 reps heavy weight, second exercise.
Sets as indicated below.

Week 1
2 pre-exhaust sets per workout:
3 workouts, 3 sets.

Week 2
3 pre-exhaust sets per workout:
3 workouts, 3 sets.

Week 3
3 pre-exhaust sets per workout:
3 workouts, 4 sets.

Week 4
3 pre-exhaust sets per workout:
3 workouts, 4 sets.

Speed of lift
1:2

Rest
Take 30 seconds between exercises and 3 minutes between pre-exhaust sets.

MONTH 11
pre-exhaust set 1

 Bench triceps dip
Targets: triceps

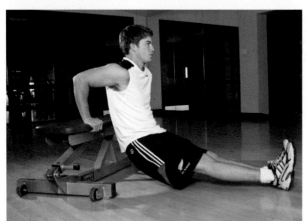 **Barbell bench press**
Targets: chest and shoulders

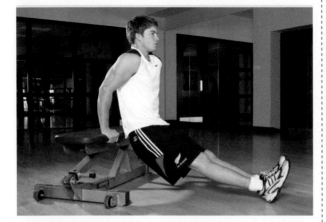

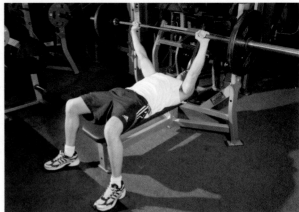

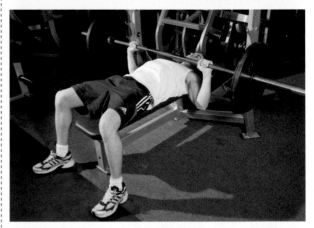

■ Grip the edge of the bench with your hands.
■ Look straight ahead.
■ Keep your legs straight, your feet together and your back upright.
■ Lower your body straight down slowly and, keeping your elbows pointing back, press back up powerfully.

■ Take bar from rack.
■ Position the bar directly above your chest with your hands wider than shoulder-width apart.
■ Ensure your head and shoulders are fully supported on the bench.
■ Maintain a natural arch in your back.
■ Keep your feet flat on floor.
■ Lower the bar to a centimetre or so above your chest then press back up powerfully without arching your back.

pre-exhaust set 2

1 Leg extension
Targets: quadriceps

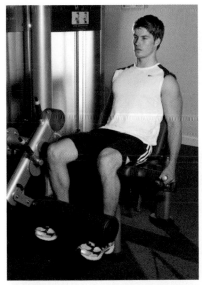

■ Sit so that your torso is angled back slightly rather than upright.
■ Look straight ahead.
■ Keep your thighs in contact with bench.

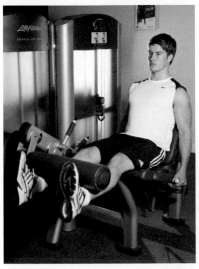

■ Squeeze your quads to lift the weight.
■ Lift to almost full extension.
■ Lower under control.
■ Keep looking forward.

2 Barbell squat
Targets: thighs and glutes

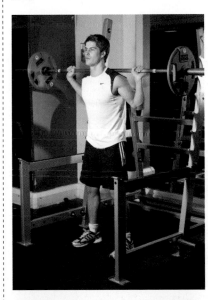

■ Take the bar from the rack and rest it across the fleshy part of your shoulders.
■ Feet shoulder-width apart.
■ Keep looking forward.
■ Keep your elbows back and brace your core.

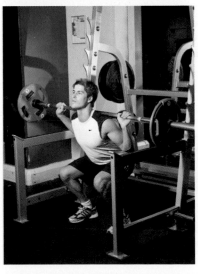

■ Lower until your thighs are parallel to the ground.
■ Maintain a natural arch in your spine.
■ Push back up through your heels.

MONTH 11
pre-exhaust set 3

1 Dumb-bell lateral raise
Targets: middle deltoids

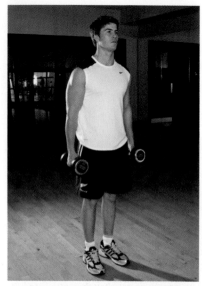

■ Look straight ahead.
■ Keep your body upright, core braced.
■ Hold dumb-bells by your sides, palms facing in.

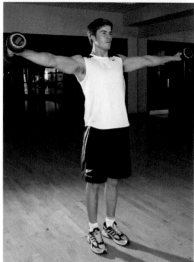

■ Lift to shoulder height.
■ Keep your core braced.
■ Look straight ahead.
■ Control weights down.

2 One-arm dumb-bell overhead press
Targets: shoulders

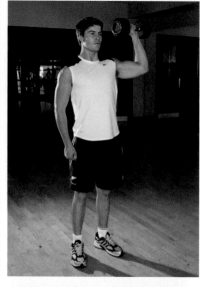

■ Look forward and brace your core.
■ Keep your right arm by your side.
■ Hold the dumb-bell in your left hand parallel to the ground.

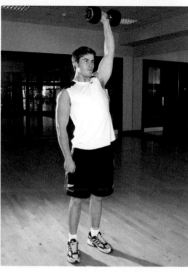

■ Press the dumb-bell up.
■ Stabilise the movement by bracing your core.
■ Control the weight down.
■ Repeat holding the dumb-bell in your opposite hand.

pre-exhaust set 4

1 Leg curl
Targets: hamstrings

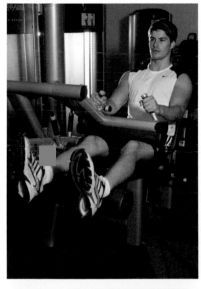

■ Adjust seat so you are sitting upright or slightly back.
■ Brace your core.
■ Look straight ahead.

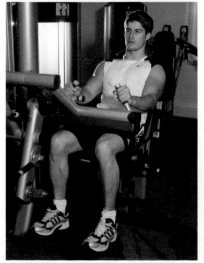

■ Pull the pad towards you.
■ Feel the tension in your hamstrings when returning weights to the start.

2 Leg press
Targets: thighs and glutes

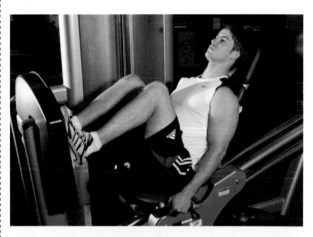

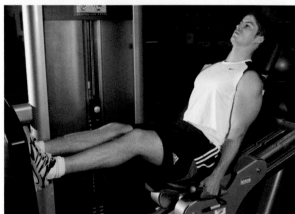

■ Push through both legs equally.
■ Extend your legs until they're nearly straight.

■ Control the weights back
■ Stop at a 90° angle at the knee.

MONTH 11
pre-exhaust set 5

 Single leg squat
Targets: thighs

 Barbell front squat
Targets: thighs and glutes

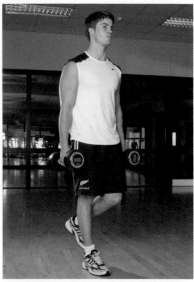

■ Hold dumbbells by sides.
■ Lift one foot off the floor slightly.
■ Keep chest up.
■ Look forward.

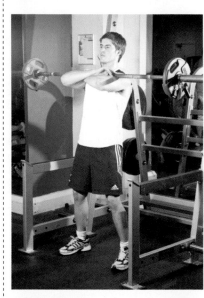

■ Take the bar from rack and rest it across your shoulders.
■ Keep upper arms parallel to the floor.
■ Maintain the natural curves of your spine.
■ Feet just beyond hip-width apart and keep looking forward.

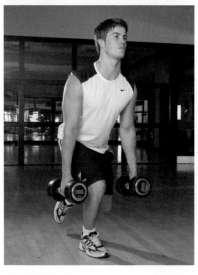

■ Keep your heel on the ground.
■ Lower until your thigh is parallel to the ground or until you break form.
■ Keep knee in line with toes.

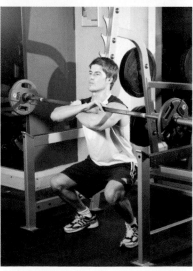

■ Lower until your thighs are parallel to the ground.
■ Push back up through your heels.
■ Keep looking forward.
■ Maintain the natural curves of your spine.

core exercises

1 Plank
Targets: core

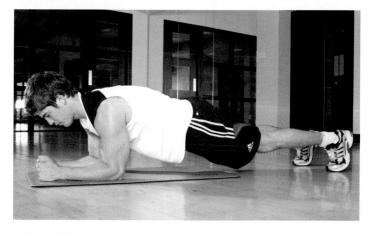

- Look down.
- Hold your body in a straight line from head to heels.
- Place your elbows beneath your shoulders.

2 Crunch
Targets: abdominals

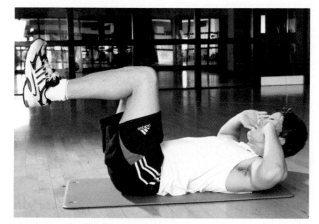 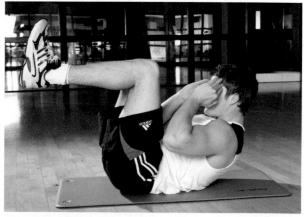

- Line your elbows up with your ears.
- Touch your fingertips to your temples.

- Contract your abdominals to lift your torso.
- Don't lift too high.
- Lower your torso under control.

Meal plan

This 42-meal plan packs in calories to help you get bigger and stronger

	Monday	Tuesday	Wednesday	Thursday
Breakfast	*Energiser smoothie* ■ Blend 2 apples, 1 stick of celery, 1 banana, 3 dates, ½tsp honey and 25g whey protein with 200-300ml water.	■ 4 scrambled egg whites on 2 slices of wholemeal toast. ■ Glass of orange juice.	■ 4 scrambled egg whites on 2 slices of wholemeal toast. ■ Glass of orange juice.	■ Porridge made with 45g oats, 300ml skimmed milk, 1tsp honey and 25g whey protein.
Morning snack	■ 1 mashed banana with 2tbsp peanut butter on 2 slices of wholemeal toast.	■ Mixed nuts, raisins and dried cranberries.	■ 120g low-fat yoghurt with blueberries, honey and oats. ■ 1 protein bar.	■ 90g mackerel on 2 slices of wholemeal toast. ■ Glass of skimmed milk.
Lunch	■ Turkey, cheese and mustard bagel. ■ 1 apple.	■ Turkey and cheese bagel. ■ 1 orange.	■ Chicken, bacon and avocado baguette. ■ 1 pear.	■ Large jacket potato with tuna, baked beans and grated cheese.
Afternoon snack	■ 1 tin of tuna with beetroot and cottage cheese.	■ Smoothie: blend 25g whey protein, 80g raspberries, 80g blueberries and 50g blackberries with 200-300ml water.	■ Smoothie: blend 25g whey protein, 100g strawberries and ½ banana with 300ml skimmed milk and 1tsp flaxseed oil.	■ Smoothie: blend 25g whey protein, 80g raspberries, 80g blueberries and 50g blackberries with 200-300ml water.
Dinner	■ 200g chicken and vegetable stir fry with red and green peppers, cashew nuts, sesame oil and seeds. ■ 70g brown rice.	■ 120g salmon with stir-fried broccoli, green beans, red peppers and spinach with sesame oil and seeds. ■ 70g brown rice.	■ 120g tuna steak with stir-fried broccoli, cashew nuts, green beans and spinach with sesame oil and seeds. ■ 70g brown rice.	■ 90g wholemeal pasta and 200g grilled chicken with jar of tomato sauce and chopped onion.
Bedtime snack	■ Smoothie: blend 25g whey protein, 80g raspberries, 80g blueberries and 50g blackberries with 200-300ml water.	■ Smoothie: blend 25g whey protein, 50g blueberries, 50g blackberries and ½ banana with 300ml skimmed milk.	■ 30g bran with sultanas and 200ml skimmed milk.	■ 120g low-fat yoghurt with strawberries.
Daily totals	■ 2,911 calories ■ 193g protein ■ 357g carbs ■ 68g fat	■ 2,857 calories ■ 196g protein ■ 345g carbs ■ 66g fat	■ 2,920 calories ■ 198g protein ■ 365g carbs ■ 68g fat	■ 2,945 calories ■ 206g protein ■ 367g carbs ■ 69g fat

Friday	Saturday	Sunday
■ Porridge made with 45g oats, 300ml skimmed milk, 1tsp honey and 25g whey protein.	■ Smoothie: blend 25g whey protein, 1 mango, 2tbsp yoghurt, 80g blueberries and 1tbsp oats with 100ml apple juice and 100ml water.	■ 2 scrambled eggs on 2 slices of wholemeal toast. ■ Glass of orange juice.
■ 1 mashed banana on 1 slice of wholemeal toast.	■ 90g sardines with lemon juice on 2 slices wholemeal toast.	■ 30g brazil nuts. ■ Glass of skimmed milk.
■ Turkey salad sandwich on wholemeal bread. ■ 1 orange.	■ Large jacket potato with baked beans and cottage cheese.	■ Large jacket potato with baked beans, tuna and grated cheese.
■ Mixed nuts, raisins and dried cranberries with cottage cheese.	■ 140g grilled chicken with beetroot.	■ Smoothie: blend 25g whey protein, 100g strawberries, ½ banana with 300ml skimmed milk and 1tsp flaxseed oil.
Chicken fajitas	■ 120g fillet steak with mashed potato and spinach.	■ 150g roast lamb with 100g new potatoes, and mixed vegetables.
■ Smoothie: blend 25g whey protein, 50g blueberries, 50g blackberries and ½ banana with 300ml skimmed milk.	■ Smoothie: blend 25g whey protein, 80g raspberries, 80g blueberries and 50g blackberries with 200-300ml water.	■ 100g cottage cheese. ■ 1 pear.
2,919 calories **203g protein** **363g carbs** **64g fat**	**2,943 calories** **212g protein** **365g carbs** **69g fat**	**3,015 calories** **208g protein** **367g carbs** **74g fat**

Chicken fajitas

serves 2

Ingredients
4 chicken breasts,
1 onion, sliced
1 green pepper, sliced
1 red pepper, sliced
Fajita mix
4 small flour tortillas
Cheddar cheese, grated
Sour cream
Guacamole
Salsa

To make
Cut chicken into strips and fry until browned, add peppers, onion and fajita mix and fry for a further 5-7mins. Serve in heated tortillas with sour cream, guacamole, salsa and grated cheese.

Workout log: month 11

See for sets, reps and times

Theme: Pre-exhaust shock tactics and unilateral movements   **Date:** _____
System: Pre-exhaust
Speed of lift: 1:2
Rest: 30 seconds between exercises and 3 minutes between pre-exhaust sets

Exercise	Sets	Reps/Time	Weight
Select 2-3 pre-exhaust sets per workout that work different body parts			
Bench triceps dip			N/A
Barbell bench press			
Leg extension			
Barbell squat			
Dumb-bell lateral raise			
One-arm dumb-bell overhead press			
Leg curl			
Leg press			
Single leg squat			
Barbell front squat			
Plank			N/A
Crunch			N/A

Cardio record your sessions below

Workout comments:

Self tests (see p36)

Record your performance below to monitor your progress

Plank endurance

seconds

Lying hamstring stretch

seconds

Press-up

number

Vertical jump

height

Strength

bench kilograms

squat kilograms

(other)

(other)

Measure up

chest

shoulders

thighs

calves

biceps/triceps

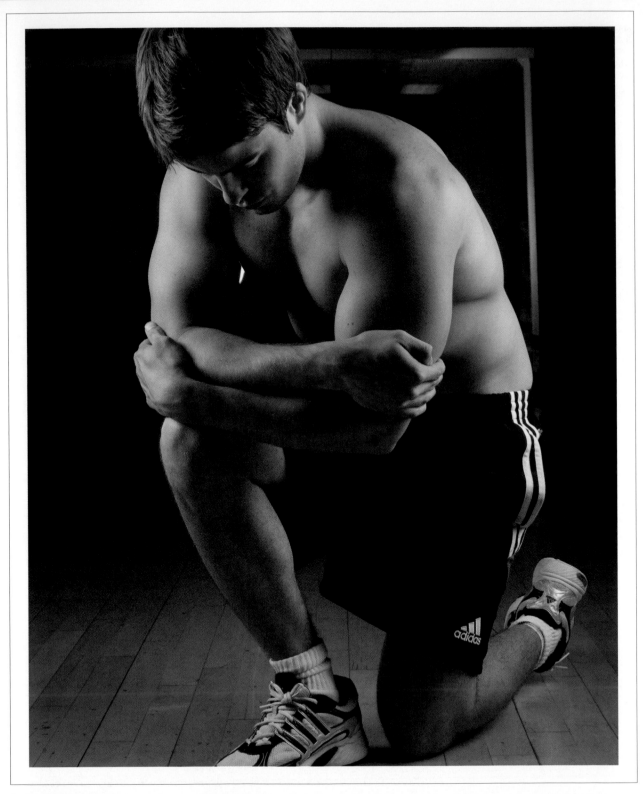

Ultimate Workout Plan
MONTH 12

You've reached the end of the *Ultimate Workout Plan* – well almost. By now you should have packed on a substantial amount of lean muscle and will have developed a great physique. This last month is all about adding the final touches. You'll lift light to heavy weights, with high repetitions to pump, grow and tone – using a decreasing load pyramid. The cardio workouts will contribute to your fat burning and remove that final layer of body fat to reveal your new cover-model body.

A decreasing load pyramid will allow you to increase the number of reps as you work 'down' through the sets. Because the first set is heavy you must be mentally focussed to tackle it.

'This month is all about adding the final touches'

Month 12:
The finishing touches

System
Pyramid, with decreasing load

Bodyweight
Hanging straight-leg lift
3 x 15
1 minute recovery between sets.
Crunch with twist
3 x 20
1 minute recovery between sets.

Free weights
Barbell squat
Barbell split squat
Barbell shoulder press
Barbell bench press
Barbell deadlift (1:2 speed)
Barbell high pull
Barbell front squat (1:2 speed)
Dumb-bell flyes
Barbell step-up

Fixed weights
Lat pull-down (1:2 speed)

Cardio
2 x complementary interval cardiovascular workouts (see p28).

Workouts
For each workout, select six exercises that work different body parts.
Do three workouts a week.

Weeks 1-4
1 x 3 heavy weight
1 x 5 medium-heavy weight
1 x 12 medium weight
2 x 20-25 light weight

You must push to fatigue on the heavy pyramid set. If you have a training partner you could attempt some forced reps (see page 19).

Speed
1:1 (unless otherwise indicated)

Rest
2 minutes between heavy and medium-heavy sets and exercises, and 1 minute between other sets and exercises.

MONTH 12
workout

 ## Barbell squat
Targets: thighs and glutes

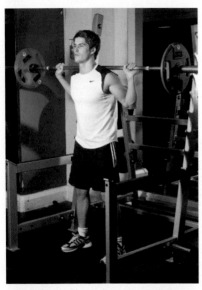

- Take the bar from the rack and rest it across the fleshy part of your shoulders.
- Keep your elbows back and your core braced.
- Feet shoulder-width apart.

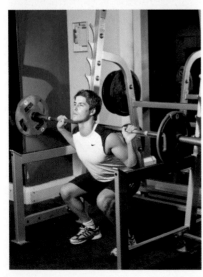

- Keep looking forward.
- Lower until your thighs are parallel to the ground.
- Maintain a natural arch in your back.
- Push back up through your heels.

2 Barbell split squat
Targets: thighs and glutes

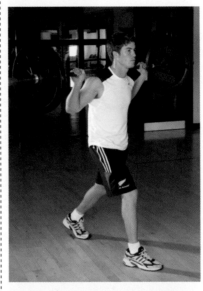

- Support the bar on the fleshy part of your shoulders.
- Look straight ahead and take a large step forward.
- Brace your core and keep your knee in line with your toes.

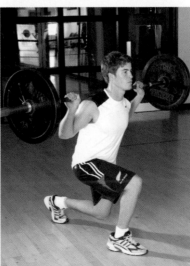

- Support weight on toes of rear foot.
- Maintain a natural arch in your back.
- Lower until your front thigh is parallel to the ground or until you break form.

Barbell shoulder press
Targets: deltoids

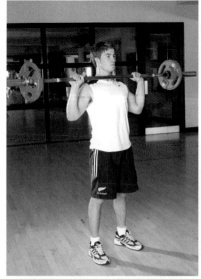

■ Brace your core.
■ Keep feet shoulder-width apart.
■ Look forward.
■ Hold the bar on your upper chest.

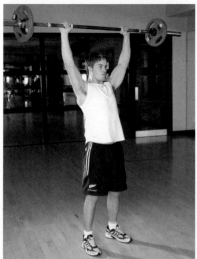

■ Press the bar directly overhead.
■ Keep your core braced and don't tilt your hips forward.

4 **Barbell bench press**
Targets: pecs, deltoids and triceps

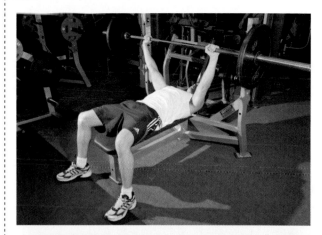

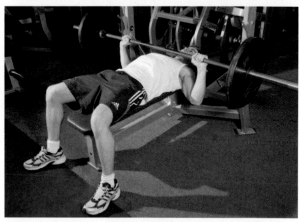

■ Take the bar from the rack.
■ Position the bar directly above your chest with hands wider than shoulder-width apart.
■ Ensure your head and shoulders are fully supported on the bench.

■ Maintian a natural arch in your back.
■ Keep your feet flat on the floor.
■ Lower the bar to a centimetre or so above your chest then press back up powerfully without arching your back.

MONTH 12
workout

5 Barbell deadlift

SPEED 1:2

Targets: back and hamstrings

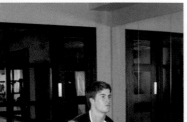

■ Look straight ahead, with your shoulders back and brace your core.
■ Keep your shoulders over the bar and keep the bar close to your shins.
■ Maintain the natural curves of your back.
■ Keep your feet shoulder-width apart.
■ Hold the bar with a grip that's slightly wider than shoulder width.

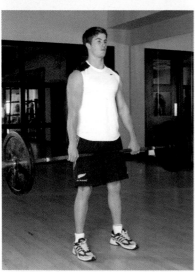

■ Start the lift by pullig with your glutes.
■ Push up through your heels, keeping the bar close to your shins.
■ As the bar passes your knees, push your hips forward.

6 Barbell high pull

Targets: legs, glutes, back, shoulders

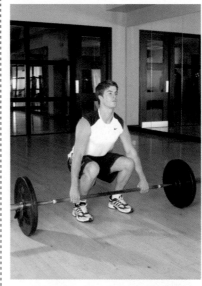

■ Place your feet shoulder-width apart.
■ Hold the bar with a grip that's slightly wider than shoulder width using an overhand grip.
■ Keep your heels on the floor and your arms long.
■ Lean slightly back.
■ Drive up through the legs.
■ When the bar reaches hip level, push your hips forward.

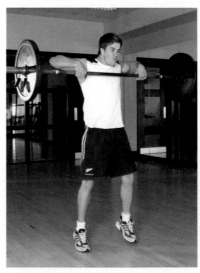

■ Pull the bar up with your arms.
■ Extend onto toes.
■ Pull bar to shoulder height.
■ Control the bar back to start position.

Lat pull-down
Targets: lats and upper back

 SPEED 1:2

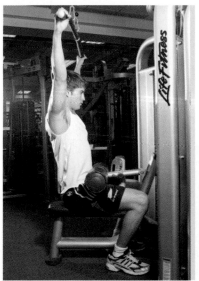

■ Take a wide grip on the bar.
■ Retract your shoulder blades and keep your torso upright.
■ Adjust the pad so it sits snugly on your thighs to minimise movement.

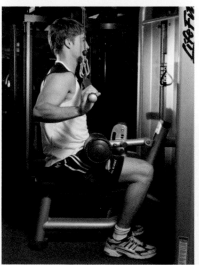

■ Pull the bar down in front of your upper chest and squeeze your lats at the bottom of the move.
■ Resist the temptation to lean back too far to aid the movement.

8 **Barbell front squat**
Targets: thighs and glutes – throws emphasis onto quads

SPEED 1:2

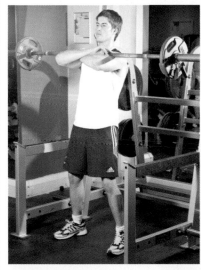

■ Take the bar from the rack and rest it across the front of your shoulders.
■ Grip the bar with your fingertips and keep your upper arms parallel to the floor.
■ Feet shoulder-width apart.

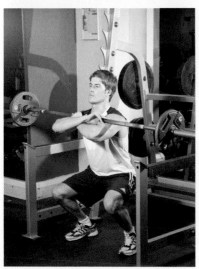

■ Lower until your thighs are parallel to the ground.
■ Push back up through your heels.
■ Keep looking forward.

MONTH 12
workout

9 Dumb-bell flye
Targets: chest

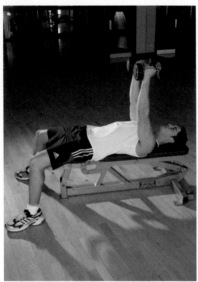

■ Hold dumb-bells directly above chest with palms facing each other.
■ Keep your feet flat on the floor.
■ Support your head and shoulders on bench.

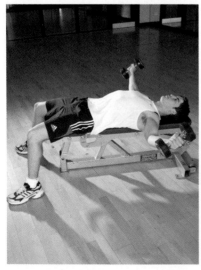

■ Lower the dumb-bells in an arc out to the sides.
■ Lower the dumb-bells as far as is comfortable, keeping a slight bend in your elbows.
■ Use your pectorial muscles to reverse the movement back to the start.
■ Don't arch your back.

10 Barbell step-up
Targets: thighs and glutes

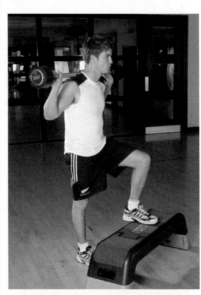

■ Look straight ahead.
■ Rest bar across the fleshy part of shoulders.
■ Use a bench or step that's no higher than knee height.
■ Place your left foot firmly on the step.

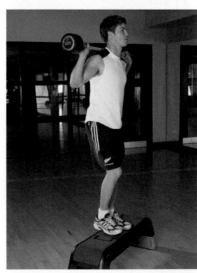

■ Push up through your left leg.
■ Keep your back upright.
■ Bring right leg up to join the left leg.
■ Step back down with your right leg.
■ Step up again, this time with your right foot, and then continue to alternate legs.

11 ▸ Hanging straight leg lift
Targets: abdominals and hip flexors

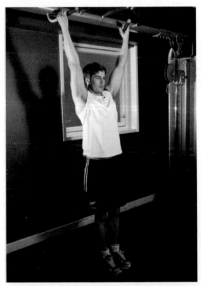

- Hang from bar.
- Steady your body, don't swing.
- Look straight ahead.

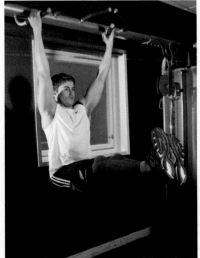

- Brace your core.
- Lift your legs without swining and lower under control.

12 ▸ Crunch with twist
Targets: abdominals

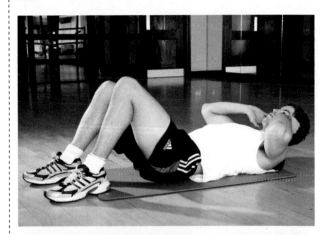

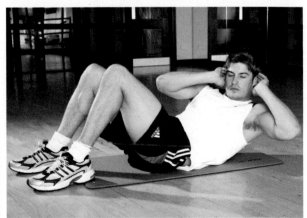

- Place fingers by ears, elbows back.
- Feet flat on the floor.
- Keep your knees at a 90° angle.
- Contract your abs to lift your

shoulders off the floor.
- Curl your chest towards your knees and rotate your right elbow across to your left knee.
- Lower under control.
- Repeat on the other side.

Meal plan

Eat your way to the body you've always wanted with this healthy meal plan

	Monday	**Tuesday**	**Wednesday**	**Thursday**
Breakfast	■ 2 scrambled eggs and baked beans on 2 slices of wholemeal toast. ■ Glass of orange juice.	■ Porridge made with 45g oats, 300ml skimmed milk, 1tsp of honey and 25g whey protein.	■ 4 scrambled egg whites on 2 slices of wholemeal toast. ■ Glass of orange juice.	■ 45g oats with 300ml skimmed milk, 1tsp of honey and 25g whey protein.
Morning snack	■ 120g low-fat yoghurt with blueberries, honey and oats. ■ 1 protein bar.	■ 1 mashed banana on 1 slice of wholemeal toast.	■ Mixed nuts, raisins and dried cranberries.	■ 90g mackerel on 2 slices wholemeal toast. ■ Glass of skimmed milk.
Lunch	■ Chicken, bacon and avocado baguette. ■ 1 pear.	■ Turkey salad sandwich on wholemeal bread. ■ 1 orange.	■ Turkey and cheese bagel. ■ 1 orange.	■ Large jacket potato with tuna, baked beans and grated cheese.
Afternoon snack	■ Smoothie: blend 25g whey protein, 100g and ½ banana with 300ml skimmed milk and 1tsp flaxseed oil.	■ Mixed nuts, raisins and dried cranberries with cottage cheese.	Protein power smoothie ■ Blend 25g whey protein, 3 almonds, 3 brazil nuts, 80g blueberries, 2 dates, 50g natural yoghurt and ½ banana with 250ml skimmed milk. Serve chilled.	■ Smoothie: blend 25g whey protein, 80g raspberries, 80g blueberries and 50g blackberries with 200-300ml water.
Dinner	■ 120g tuna steak with stir-fried broccoli, green beans and spinach with sesame oil and seeds. ■ 70g brown rice	Beef chilli	■ 120g salmon with stir-fried broccoli, green beans, red peppers and spinach with sesame oil and seeds. ■ 70g brown rice.	■ Omelette with ham, feta cheese, olives, tomato and onion.
Bedtime snack	■ 100g cottage cheese and pineapple.	■ Smoothie: blend 25g protein, 50g blueberries, 50g blackberries, ½ banana with 300ml skimmed milk.	■ Smoothie: blend 25g whey protein, 50g blueberries, 50g blackberries, ½ banana with 300ml skimmed milk.	■ 120g low-fat yoghurt with strawberries.
Daily totals	■ 2,912 calories ■ 197g protein ■ 365g carbs ■ 67g fat	■ 2,895 calories ■ 204g protein ■ 363g carbs ■ 65g fat	■ 2,887 calories ■ 199g protein ■ 345g carbs ■ 70g fat	■ 2,954 calories ■ 205g protein ■ 367g carbs ■ 69g fat

Friday	**Saturday**	**Sunday**
■ Porridge made with 45g oats, 300ml skimmed milk, 1tsp honey, handful of blueberries and 25g whey protein.	■ Smoothie: blend 25g whey protein, 1 mango, 80g blueberries, 2tbsp natural yoghurt and 1tbsp oats with 100ml apple juice and 100ml water.	■ 2 scrambled eggs on 2 slices of wholemeal toast. ■ Glass of orange juice.
■ 1 mashed banana with 2tbsp peanut butter on 2 slices of wholemeal toast.	■ 90g sardines with lemon juice on 2 slices of wholemeal toast.	■ 30g brazil nuts. ■ Glass of skimmed milk.
■ Turkey, cheese and mustard bagel. ■ 1 apple.	■ Large jacket potato with baked beans and cottage cheese.	■ Large jacket potato with baked beans, tuna and grated cheese.
■ 1 tin of tuna with beetroot and cottage cheese.	■ 140g grilled chicken with beetroot.	■ Smoothie: blend 25g whey protein, 100g strawberries and ½ banana with 300ml skimmed milk and 1tsp flaxseed oil.
■ 120g fillet steak with mashed potato and spinach. ■ Fruit sorbet.	■ 200g chicken and vegetable stir fry with red and green peppers, cashew nuts, sesame oil and seeds. ■ 70g brown rice.	■ 150g roast beef with 100g new potatoes, and mixed vegetables.
■ Smoothie: blend 25g whey protein, 80g raspberries, 80g blueberries and 50g blackberries with 200-300ml water.	■ Smoothie: blend 25g whey protein, 80g raspberries, 80g blueberries and 50g blackberries with 200-300ml water.	■ 100g cottage cheese. ■ 1 apple.
■ 2,950 calories ■ 208g protein ■ 359g carbs ■ 68g fat	■ 2,903 calories ■ 198g protein ■ 365g carbs ■ 69g fat	■ 3,012 calories ■ 208g protein ■ 367g carbs ■ 73g fat

Beef chilli

serves 2

Ingredients
300g lean, minced beef
1 tin (400g) red kidney beans
1 tin (400g) peeled plum tomatoes
1 onion, chopped
2 cloves garlic, finely chopped
1tsp olive oil
1tsp diced chilli
1tbsp tomato purée
1tsp dried oregano
1tbsp cumin
200ml beef stock
Salt and pepper, for seasoning

To make
Fry the onion and garlic in the olive oil until soft. Add the minced beef and fry until browned. Mix in the minced chilli and stir through. Cover and simmer for 3 minutes then add the tomato purée and tinned tomatoes and simmer for further 20 minutes. Add the kidney beans, oregano, cumin and beef stock and simmer for a further 10 minutes. Season with salt and pepper to taste and serve with 70g brown rice.

Workout log: month 12

See p173 for sets, reps and times

Theme: The finishing touches
System: Pyramid with decreasing load
Speed of lift: 1:1 (except for deadlift, lat pull-down and front squat which are 1:2)
Rest: 2 minutes between heavy/medium-heavy sets and exercises and 1 minute others

Date: _____

Exercise	Sets	Reps/Time	Weight
Select 6 exercises that work different body parts			
Barbell squat			
Barbell spilt squat			
Standing barbell shoulder press			
Barbell bench press			
Barbell deadlift			
Barbell high pull			
Lat pull-down			
Barbell front squat			
Dumb-bell flye			
Barbell step-up			
Hanging straight leg lift			N/A
Crunch with twist			N/A

Cardio record your sessions below

Workout comments:

Self tests (see p36)

Record your performance below to monitor your progress

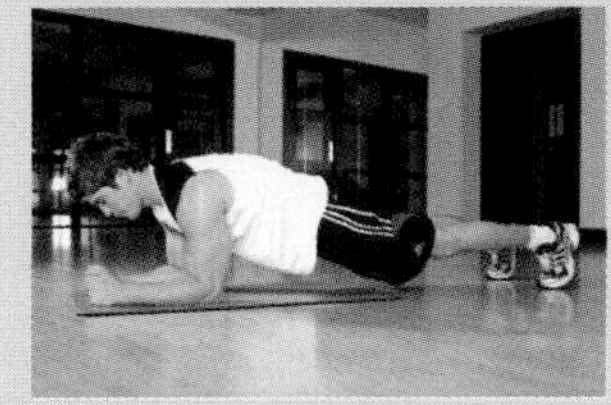

Plank endurance

seconds

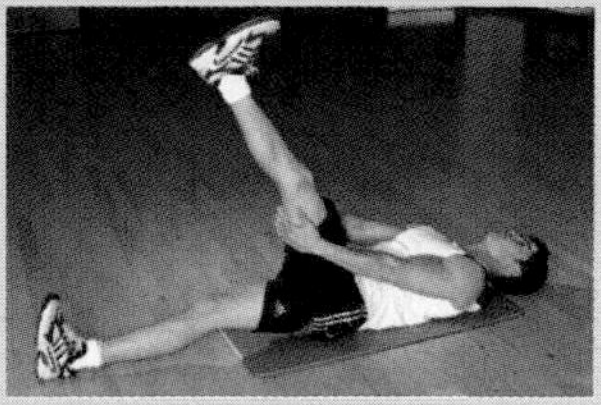

Lying hamstring stretch

seconds

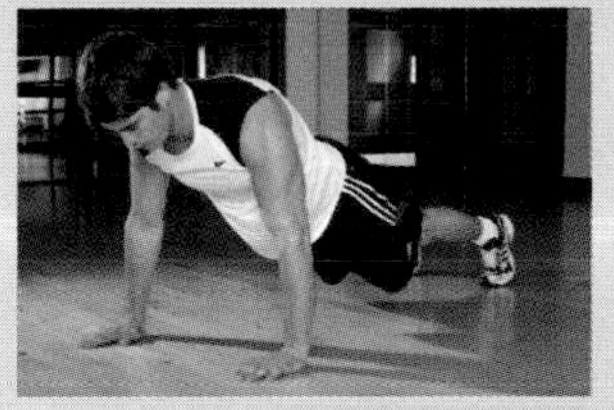

Press-up

number

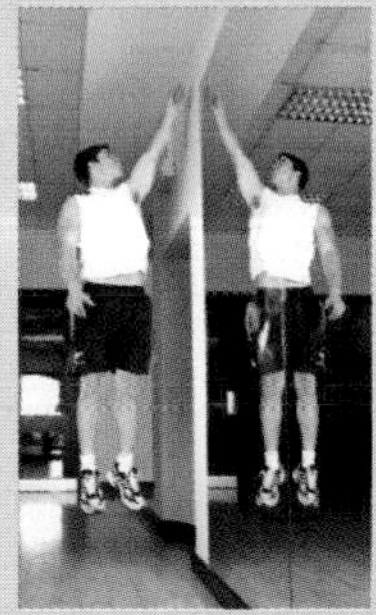

Vertical jump

height

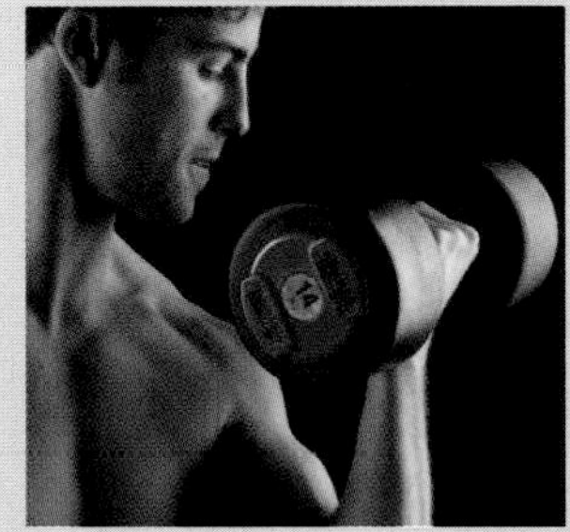

Strength

bench kilograms

squat kilograms

(other)

(other)

Measure up

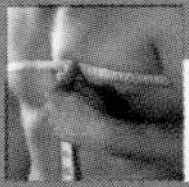

chest

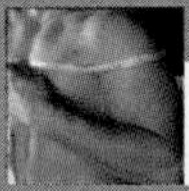

shoulders

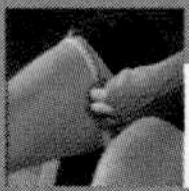

thighs

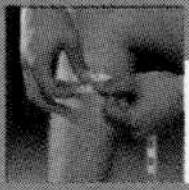

calves

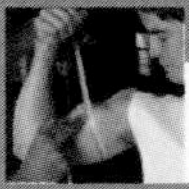

biceps/triceps

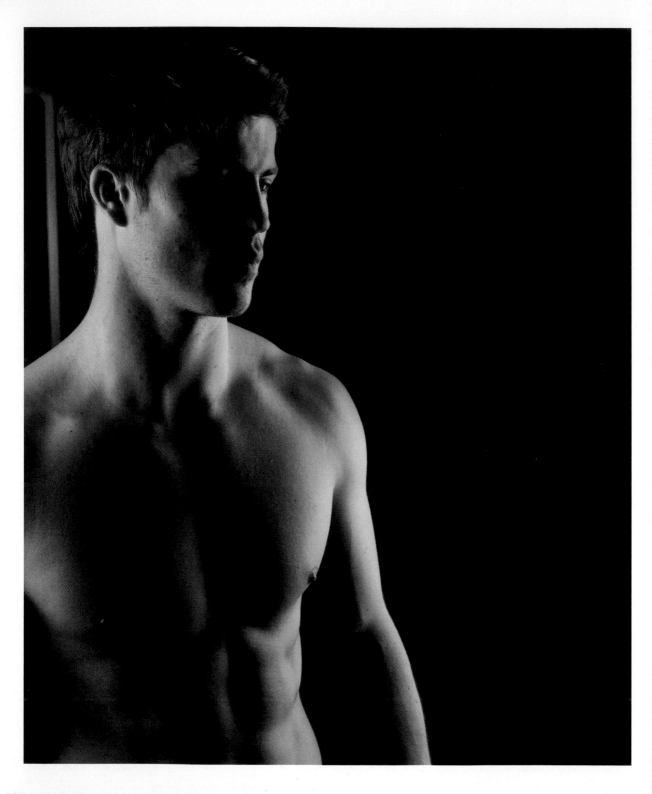

What's next?

It may be the end of the book, but the training doesn't have to stop here

Congratulations, you've reached the end of the *Ultimate Workout Plan*. By now you'll have developed a fantastic looking body, that not only attracts the admiring glances of the women you meet, but is also powerful and athletic. So, what now?

MAINTAIN

You can put your feet up for a bit if you like. Maintaining your new look will be a whole lot easier than creating it in the first place. But don't just sit back and do nothing for too long. You'll need to stay fairly active – two workouts a week should be enough – and make some adjustments to your calorie consumption to keep your body looking good. You can't simply wind down your workouts and then expect to replace the hours you once spent in the gym with hours slumped on the sofa pigging out on pizza. If you cut down on your gym sessions, you'll also need to cut down your calories or you'll soon see that six-pack disappear under an expanding beer belly.

START AGAIN!

If your new physique doesn't live up to your dream body, and you want to get even bigger, stronger and more powerful, then starting the programme again could do the trick. Make sure you

'Maintaining your new look will be easier than creating it'

give yourself a two to three week break and then start back at the beginning. It won't be quite the beginning because of the gains you've already made. You'll be starting at a higher level than before, and so you'll be able to select heavier weights for each workout than you did first time round, giving you increased overload and greater gains.

You'll also know which specific workouts work best for you. So, if you found that negative reps boosted your strength and size to a greater extent than power workouts, then you could load your programme towards negative reps. It's OK to adapt the programme slightly, as no two men will respond to the same workout in exactly the same way, but you still need to maintain balance. Don't think that because a particular workout gave you great results that you should do it all the time. If you do, you'll soon reach a training plateau and might even find that your strength and size gains start to reverse. Instead, use this guide as a template, keep varying your workouts, and you'll be well on your way to achieving the body you've always wanted. ∎

Do something different but just as challenging...

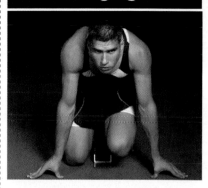

If you don't want to return to the gym full time, why not test your new physique with a sport? The programme will have given you a good idea of your body's strengths and weaknesses, and therefore which sports will suit you best. For example:

Scored excellent, or above, on the power test, bench press and squat. Try: **rugby**

Scored excellent, or above, on the press-up endurance test; excellent, or above, on the squat and bench press; and excellent, or above, on the power test. Try: **sprinting**

Scored excellent on the plank and press-up muscular endurance tests, good-to-excellent on the squat and bench press. Try: **climbing**

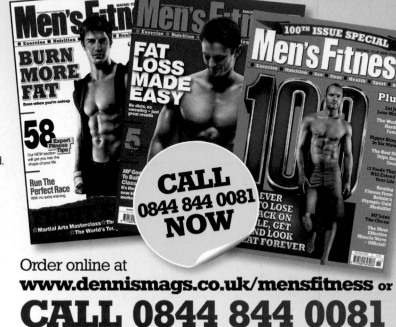